Childbed Fever

With a new introduction by the authors

K. Codell Carter
Barbara R. Carter

Childbed Fever

A Scientific Biography of Ignaz Semmelweis

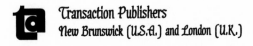
Transaction Publishers
New Brunswick (U.S.A.) and London (U.K.)

Library of Congress Catalog Number: 2004056156
ISBN: 1-4128-0467-1
Printed in the United States of America

Library of Congress Cataloging-in-Publication Data

Carter, K. Codell (Kay Codell), 1939-
    Childbed fever : a scientific biography of Ignaz Semmelweis / K. Codell Carter and Barbara R. Carter.
        p. cm.
    Previously published in 1994 by Greenwood Press.
    Includes bibliographical references and index.
    ISBN 1-4128-0467-1 (pbk. : alk. paper)
        1. Semmelweis, Ignâc Fèlèp, 1818-1865. 2. Obstetricians—Hungary—Biography. 3. Puerperal septicemia—History. I. Carter, Barbara R. II. Title.

RG510.S4C37   2004
618.2'0092—dc22
[B]   2004056156

Copyright Acknowledgments

Excerpts from *The Etiology, Concept, and Prophylaxis of Childbed Fever,* ed. and trans. by K. Codell Carter (Madison: The University of Wisconsin Press; © 1983 by the Board of Regents of The University of Wisconsin System).

Excerpts from K. Codell Carter, "Ignaz Semmelweis, Carl Mayrhofer, and the Rise of Germ Theory," *Medical History* 29 (1985): 33-53; and K. Codell Carter, "Semmelweis and His Predecessors," *Medical History* 25 (1981): 57-72. Copyright the Trustees of the Wellcome Trust, and reproduced with their permission.

Contents

Transaction Introduction

We know of no story more engaging and moving than the life and work of Ignaz Semmelweis. In writing this book, our goal was to make the Semmelweis story available to a general audience; unfortunately the book appeared only in an expensive library edition. During the decade since its first publication, hoping to bring the story to more readers, we considered publishing the book, privately, in an inexpensive paperback format. Now, because Transaction Publishers has kindly invited us to reissue the book, we have new hope that our goal may yet be attained.

Parts of Semmelweis's story have been told before. His work is the subject of more than the usual number of scholarly books and articles. Morton Thompson's 1949 fictionalized account of his life and work, *The Cry and the Covenant*, sold over a million copies. Sherwin B. Nuland's *The Doctors' Plague: Germs, Childbed Fever, and the Strange Story of Ignác Semmelweis* appeared in 2003. However, few authors have made the necessary effort to understand (much less to explain) the system of ideas to which Semmelweis was drawn. As a result, while the pathos of Semmelweis's life comes through in virtually every account, almost no one, not even Nuland, grasps Semmelweis's significance in the history of medicine. We find our book to be better written and more engaging than any of the other accounts, but an even more important virtue is that it alone makes clear exactly why Semmelweis was so important. His contribution was different from and more profound than one would infer from any other published account of his life and work.

In 1846 Vienna, as what would now be called a head resident of obstetrics, Semmelweis confronted the terrible reality of childbed fever. This disease struck post partum women within twenty-four to forty-eight hours after delivery and killed prodigious numbers of women throughout Europe and America. In some maternity clinics, through several decades, the mortality rate exceeded twenty percent. In some hospitals, over a period of weeks, epidemics of childbed fever killed seventy percent or more of all the women who gave birth. In Vienna, the mortality rate averaged a relatively benign ten percent, but even at that comparatively low rate, more than 2000 women died each year from the disease. All told, in nineteenth-century Europe, childbed fever killed more than a million women.

In May 1847, Semmelweis was struck by the realization that the diseased women in his clinic had all been infected by decaying remains of human tissues. Infection occurred because medical personnel did not wash their hands thoroughly after conducting autopsies in the morgue. He immediately began requiring everyone working in his clinic to wash in a chlorine solution. The mortality rate immediately fell to about one percent. Over the next two years, Semmelweis refined his understanding of childbed fever and accumulated impressive statistical evidence in support of his views. By 1850 he was convinced that *every* case of childbed fever was due to what he described as the resorption of decaying organic matter.

While some of Semmelweis's contemporaries were willing to try chlorine washings, at the time everyone rejected his claim that every case of childbed fever was due to one universal necessary cause. The idea that every case of any disease would have a single universal cause was fundamentally inconsistent with existing medical beliefs, and even his teachers and supposed friends in the Vienna medical school balked at this radical claim.

Within ten years, Semmelweis died after being beaten by the guards of an insane asylum to which he had been committed. By the time of his death, only a few physicians had accepted his account of childbed fever. However, in time his views prevailed. Within about two decades, several prominent researchers acknowledged that Semmelweis had helped provide a true understanding of childbed fever and, ultimately, of infectious diseases generally.

Semmelweis's claims were starkly inconsistent with medical theories current in the 1850s; understandably, this made his claims difficult to accept. However, by forcing physicians to abandon their cherished theories, his work led to the adoption of an entirely new way of thinking about disease. Thus, he did not simply contribute a beneficial new practice (disinfectant washings); rather he helped create an entirely new theory of disease. This new theory, sometimes referred to as the etiological standpoint, still dominates medicine today. Failure to grasp the relation between Semmelweis's work and the rise of the etiological standpoint is the main defect in the standard accounts of Semmelweis's life and work.

We are delighted to have yet another opportunity to make this clear.

Finally, we would like to comment on the title of this book. The title we originally chose was *Houses of Death: An Account of Childbed Fever and of the Work of Ignaz Semmelweis*. This title was suggested by a story that is narrated in the first paragraph of the Preface (to which the reader is invited to turn). However, the initial publisher found the title too dramatic, and Transaction Publishers has elected to retain the title under which the book was originally published. As authors, we still judge our originally intended title to best reflect the content and the tone of the book.

K. Codell Carter
Barbara R. Carter

Preface

A nineteenth-century medical student overheard a senior physician say that charity maternity clinics—birth houses, as they were called—were really houses of death. He was surprised by the comment and asked a hospital worker why the physician would say such a thing. "It's obvious," the worker replied; "the morgue is always full of corpses from the maternity wards, like fish on a slab."[1]

Medical advances are purchased by two kinds of sacrifice: the sacrifice of researchers trying to understand disease and the sacrifice of patients who die or are killed in the process. One striking nineteenth-century medical advance was the recognition that microorganisms cause disease. This particular advance was purchased, in part, by the sacrifice of hundreds of thousands of young women who died, following childbirth, of a terrible disease known as childbed fever—a disease that was rampant in the charity maternity clinics of the early nineteenth century.

In 1847 a young Hungarian obstetrician, Ignaz Semmelweis, discovered how the incidence of childbed fever could be significantly reduced. However, Semmelweis interpreted his discovery in a way that was inconsistent with contemporary medical doctrine, and his ideas were ridiculed and rejected by his fellow physicians. Eighteen years passed; each year, while the doctors argued, thousands more women perished in maternity clinics throughout Europe. Then, at the age of forty-two, Semmelweis died in a Viennese insane asylum after having been severely beaten by the asylum guards. In the same year, an Austrian obstetrician named Carl Mayrhofer published an essay in which he argued that childbed fever was invariably caused by microoganisms. This discovery, which was based partly on Semmelweis's work, was also rejected by many prominent obstetricians. However, a few physicians were persuaded by the evidence, and slowly the truth prevailed.

The moving and pathetic story of Ignaz Semmelweis has been told before. Yet his work is not widely known, and few of those who know of his work understand the true nature of his contribution. In writing this book, our purpose is to tell his story in a way that requires no special background in medicine or in medical history. Our hope is that more people will understand Semmelweis's work and comprehend the terrible sacrifices from which our medical system has emerged.

Many friends have helped us prepare this book. For their various contributions, we thank (in alphabetical order) Linda Hunter Adams, Diane and Travis Anderson, Carolyn and Stewart Armour, Nina and Sherman Carter, Helen Dixon, Janice and Jim Faulconer, Kent and Pat Larkin, Valerie Merit, Mark Olsen, Jan and Janice Nelson, Prascilla Hong Mee Park, Karen Pierotti, Dawn Rosquist, Susan Scott, Heather Seferovich, Jim and Julie Siebach, and Marcus Smith. We thank Josef Antall, recently deceased, previously director of the Semmelweis Institute for the History of Medicine and former Prime Minister of Hungary, for numerous enlightening conversations about the life and work of Ignaz Semmelweis. We thank Lajos Madgar for helping us locate and understand various Hungarian texts, and István Benedek for discussing with us the details of Semmelweis's death. We thank the University of Wisconsin Press for permission to use several passages from the translation of Semmelweis's *Etiology of Childbed Fever* (copyright by the Board of Regents of the University of Wisconsin System). Some of these passages have been modified slightly to bring them into accord with the terminology of this book. Two earlier essays, ''Semmelweis and His Predecessors'' and ''Ignaz Semmelweis, Carl Mayrhofer, and the Rise of Germ Theory,'' provided the basis for chapters 3, 4, and 5. These essays, which appeared originally in *Medical History*, are copyrighted by the Trustees of the Wellcome Trust and are used with their permission. Finally, we thank Brigham Young University for years of generous research support that led directly to several earlier publications and, indirectly, to this one as well.

Unless otherwise noted, the translations from all non-English sources are our own.

Wells-Next-the-Sea, Norfolk
March 1993

Note

1. Ignaz Semmelweis, *The Etiology, Concept, and Prophylaxis of Childbed Fever*, ed. and trans. K. Codell Carter (Madison: University of Wisconsin, 1983), p. 215.

1

Vienna's General Hospital

In the late eighteenth century, the Austrian Hapsburgs ruled an empire that included most of central Europe. It was a time of relative peace and prosperity. After two hundred years of intermittent struggle, Hapsburg armies had finally dislodged the Ottoman Turks from Hungary and were gradually driving them south through the Balkans. Austrian baroque architecture culminated in the rebuilding of the Danube monasteries at Melk, St. Florian, Göttweig, and Kremsmünster; Haydn and Mozart were composing in Vienna; the Enlightenment was under way. Joseph II, the most progressive and rationalistic of all the Hapsburg rulers, turned his attention to domestic problems.

At the end of the eighteenth century, about 250,000 people lived in Vienna. Contemporaries estimated that the population included between two thousand and ten thousand prostitutes and between five hundred and four thousand kept mistresses.[1] Many more thousands of single women barely survived as hod carriers, day laborers, seamstresses, cooks, chambermaids, and washerwomen. In a city never accused of moral austerity, the consequences were abortion and illegitimacy. Unwed mothers accounted for half of the live births[2]—almost twice the rate of present-day America. Poverty forced most of these women to undergo delivery in the maternity facilities of the Viennese charity hospitals, where conditions were far from satisfactory. Some charity facilities were open to the public, and the unmarried mothers were exposed to scorn and ridicule from passersby.[3] Once out of the hospitals, many indigent women were unable to support their babies, but few charitable institutions would accept and care for the newborn. This led to abandonment and infanticide—practices judged to be both immoral and contrary to the interests of the state. Joseph II attacked these problems by constructing a new hospital that provided free and humane medical care for the indigent.

During Joseph II's reign, the center of Vienna was still enclosed by enormous medieval walls although the fortifications were obsolete and the city was spreading beyond them in all directions. Not far outside the walls, on the northwest edge of the city, was a rambling, one-hundred-year-old poorhouse that was the principal residence for Vienna's orphans, invalids, aged, and infirm. In less than three years, from planning to completion, the poorhouse was rebuilt and expanded into the Viennese General Hospital. The first patients were admitted in August 1784.

The General Hospital, which remains in service today, is a short walk from the center of Vienna and is now surrounded by gray office buildings and apartment houses. However, drawings and paintings made soon after its construction show that it was originally encircled by farms and gardens. Less than a mile north of the hospital, the countryside rises toward Leopoldsberg and Kahlenberg—hills overlooking the city that, since Roman times, have been covered with vineyards and the celebrated Vienna Woods.

The General Hospital occupies a system of buildings that surrounds a dozen large rectangular courtyards arranged like an irregular checkerboard. The courtyards contain gardens, shady trees, walks, and occasional statues of prominent persons who have been associated with Viennese medicine. The hospital buildings are two and three stories high and are contiguous so that personnel can pass from one building to another without going outside. The buildings are narrow enough that some of the larger rooms overlook courtyards on two sides. Originally, the entire complex was divided in half by an imaginary axis extending straight ahead—almost due north—from the main entrance: the right side of the complex was for women, and the left for men.

The hospital was built to accommodate two thousand patients, and it began operations with a staff of only 20 physicians and 140 attendants.[4] Attendants worked twenty-four-hour shifts and while on duty slept in the same rooms as their patients.

There were three classes of accommodations: one for the indigent, who paid nothing for their care; and two classes for paying patients, in which better service was provided depending on the amount the patient was prepared to pay. Wealthy patients staying in first-class accommodations had private rooms and could be accompanied and served by their own domestic help. Charity patients occupied large rooms, most of which held about twenty beds; and these patients were expected to perform most of the ordinary housekeeping tasks for themselves.

The insane were located in a separate building called the "Fools' Tower." It more nearly resembles a fortress than a hospital facility. The building is round and five stories high; it has only one entrance. Each floor has twenty-eight cells evenly spaced around the outside wall. Each cell has one narrow window secured originally by iron bars. The circular core of the building contains facilities for attendants, round passageways on each floor providing access to the cells, and a central stairway that connects all five floors. In the eighteenth century, entering or leaving the Fools' Tower required passing through a series of heavy oak doors, each guarded by an attendant.

The idea of constructing large charity hospitals was not unique to the Hapsburgs. During the late eighteenth century, hospitals similar to the Viennese General Hospital were constructed in major cities throughout Europe. In comparison to other European institutions, however, conditions in Vienna's General Hospital were quite favorable. In 1828, the Hôtel-Dieu in Paris had 1,219 beds, of which 406 were three feet wide and 733 were four feet four inches wide. In the early nineteenth century, the number of patients in the Hôtel-Dieu ranged from two thousand to five thousand; and contemporary observers noted that there were often four, five, or even six patients in a bed.[5] In the maternity clinic at the Hôtel-Dieu, there were generally three or four patients in each bed. The pregnant and the recently delivered, the diseased and the healthy, prostitutes and married women—all were mixed together indiscriminately in the same beds. By contrast, in the Viennese General Hospital, one patient to a bed was always the rule.

What are diseases? One way to answer this question is by identifying groups of symptoms. Particular diseases can then be distinguished and characterized in terms of these symptoms. This is how diseases were generally thought of in the early nineteenth century. Mumps was a swelling in the throat, and hydrophobia (rabies) an inability to swallow, and phthisis (tuberculosis) a coughing up of blood and pus.

If several cases of a disease occurred at the same time and in the same general area, the disease was said to be "epidemic." The occurrence of an epidemic suggested that the victims may have been subjected to some noxious atmospheric influence. On the other hand, if only a few persons contracted a particular disease, the cases were called "sporadic." Sporadic cases were usually ascribed to some cause that was more or less unique to the patient; these could include heredity or even previous diseases, such as smallpox or syphilis, as well as various occupational hazards or kinds of behavior. For example, in 1825 one British physician identified the following possible causes of sporadic phthisis:

> hereditary disposition; . . . certain diseases, such as catarrh,
> pneumonic inflammation, hoemoptoe, syphilis, scrofula,

smallpox, and measles; particular employments exposing artificers to dust, such as needle-pointers, stone cutters, millers, etc.; or to the fumes of metals or minerals under a confined and unwholesome air; violent passions, exertions, or affections of the mind, as grief, disappointment, anxiety, or close application to study, without using proper exercise; playing much on wind instruments; frequent and excessive debaucheries, late watching, and drinking freely of strong liquors: great evacuations, as diarrhea, diabetes, excessive venery, fluor albus, immoderate discharge of the menstrual flux, and the continuing to suckle too long under a debilitated state; and, lastly, the application of cold, either by too quick a change of apparel, keeping on wet clothes, lying in damp beds, or exposing the body too suddenly to cool air when heated by exercise; in short, by any thing that gives a considerable check to the perspiration.[6]

Most deviations from normal life were regarded as possible causes for sporadic disease. No one entertained the idea that every case of any given disease could be due to one specific cause.

In the early nineteenth century, medical treatment was mostly the same as it had been for centuries. Physicians thought of themselves as part of a continuous and ancient tradition of medical practitioners that extended back to the ancient Romans and Greeks. And indeed most of the techniques in common use had been employed by Greek and Roman physicians more than two thousand years earlier.

Disease was often associated with fever and inflammation, and increased body heat was also observed in robust patients who ate too much. Partly because excess heat seemed to be involved both in overeating and in illness, fever and inflammation were often attacked by trying to remove the excess heat that seemed to result from the immoderate consumption of rich foods. This approach was called the "antiphlogistic regimen"; it included dietary restrictions, the use of laxatives and emetics, blistering, the application of cooling lotions, and especially bloodletting. By contrast, in other cases, disease seemed to arise because the patient was weak and undernourished or overworked. These cases required the opposite approach. Physicians tried to strengthen the patient by administering tonics and alcohol, by ensuring the consumption of nourishing foods, and by prescribing rest. This strategy was called "supportive treatment."

These commonsense ideas about disease created a practical dilemma. Many of the patients treated in the charity hospitals were undernourished and yet at the same time feverish. Fever called for the antiphlogistic regimen. But malnourished charity patients were often too weak to withstand bloodletting and seemed to require supportive treatment. The usual solution was a compromise: physicians applied supportive treatment until the patient seemed strong enough to withstand antiphlogistic measures. Then red towels were brought out, and blood was drawn. Medical writers often warned that the proper therapy could be selected only by carefully considering the details of each individual case.

Physicians believed illness more often resulted from excessive consumption than from deficiency, and the antiphlogistic regimen was more common than was supportive treatment. Bloodletting was used to treat almost every disease. One British medical text recommended bloodletting for acne, asthma, cancer, cholera, coma, convulsions, diabetes, epilepsy, gangrene, gout, herpes, indigestion, insanity, jaundice, leprosy, ophthalmia, plague, pneumonia, scurvy, smallpox, stroke, tetanus, tuberculosis, and for some one hundred other diseases. Bloodletting was even used to treat most forms of hemorrhaging such as nosebleed, excessive menstruation, or hemorrhoidal bleeding. Before surgery or at the onset of childbirth, blood was removed to prevent inflammation. Before amputation it was customary to remove a quantity of blood equal to the amount believed to circulate in the limb that was to be removed.

To treat or to prevent general or systemic symptoms like fever, blood was drawn by opening major veins or arteries. It was judged most effective to bleed patients while they were sitting upright or standing erect, and blood was often removed until the patient fainted. To treat or to prevent local inflammation, blood was removed locally by abrading or cutting the skin or by applying leeches.

When a leech is applied to some body surface, it punctures the skin with a small tooth and secretes chemicals that prevent blood coagulation. It then consumes about half an ounce of blood and drops off. The application of leeches seemed to be an ideal way to combat inflammation. Leeches were applied to any accessible inflamed body surface, including the interior of the mouth and throat, the vagina, and the rectum. Physicians often reported the simultaneous use of fifty or more leeches on a given patient, and leeches were often used together with other techniques for removing blood. Since leeches were used repeatedly and in the treatment of various diseases, it was possible for the leeches themselves to convey disease. Cases were sometimes reported in which leeches seemed to have communicated syphilis by being used first on persons who had the disease and later on other persons.[7] When leeches were placed in the mouth, they sometimes worked their way down the throat until they blocked the air passage and the patient suffocated.

Leeches became especially popular in the early nineteenth century. Through the 1830s the French imported about forty million leeches a year for medical purposes, and in the next decade, England imported six million leeches a year from France alone.[8] Through the early decades of the century, hundreds of millions of leeches were used by physicians throughout Europe.

One typical course of medical treatment began on 13 July 1824. At nine P.M., a French sergeant was stabbed through the chest while engaged in single combat; within minutes he fainted from loss of blood. He was moved to a local hospital where he was immediately bled twenty ounces to prevent inflammation. During the night he was bled another twenty-four ounces. The chief surgeon arrived early the next morning and bled the patient another ten ounces; during the next fourteen hours he was bled five more times. In the first twenty-four hours of treatment, medical attendants intentionally removed more than half of this patient's normal supply of about ten pints of blood. Bleedings continued over the next several days. By 29 July the wound had become inflamed. The physician applied thirty-two leeches to the most sensitive part of the wound. Over the next three days there were more bleedings and a total of forty more leeches. The sergeant recovered and was discharged on 3 October. His physician wrote that "by the large quantity of blood lost, amounting to 170 ounces [nearly eleven pints], besides that drawn by the application of leeches [perhaps another two pints], the life of the patient was preserved."[9] By ninteenth-century standards, thirteen pints of blood taken over the space of a month was a large but not an exceptional quantity. The medical literature of the period contains many similar accounts—some successful, some not.

In addition to the antiphlogistic regimen and supportive treatment, physicians prescribed numerous medications. Three especially popular drugs were mercury (usually in a compound called "calomel"), antimony (usually called "emetic tartar"), and arsenic. All three were toxic and were prescribed in potentially lethal doses. Especially in treating life-threatening diseases, physicians believed that administering drugs or removing blood could be effective only when performed on a scale that would itself endanger the life of the patient; such procedures were called "heroic therapies."

Surgical treatment was especially perilous to patients. There was no effective anesthetic; patients were simply tied down, a small block of wood was placed between their teeth, and the surgeon began cutting. The pain and shock of surgical procedures were often fatal. At the time, no one saw any reason for sterile operating conditions. Surgeons usually worked wearing blood-stained aprons over their ordinary street clothing. Blood encrusted clothing was regarded as a sign of the wide experience of the surgeon. Between operations, instruments were merely rinsed in tap water or not cleaned at all. Some surgeons were offended at the suggestion that they should wash their hands prior to surgery; they felt that their social status as gentlemen was inconsistent with the idea that their hands could be unclean. Surgical incisions were usually packed with common lint and then bandaged. However, at Vienna's General Hospital, the preferred treatment was to cover the incision with wet sponges and then rinse it frequently with cold tap water. As we now know, both procedures were conducive to infection. Not surprisingly, less than half of all surgical patients survived.

After surgery, patients risked catching various diseases. Among the most common was surgical fever—pain, inflammation, and a high temperature. Many patients contracted erysipelas, a painful inflammation that spread rapidly through the skin and sub-cutaneous tissues. Another problem was blood poisoning, in which the victim's blood seemed itself to degenerate; blood poisoning was classified either as septicemia or as pyemia depending on the amount and kind of pus that appeared in the blood. There was also hospital gangrene, a particularly loathsome disorder in which all the tissues slowly but inevitably decomposed while giving off a noisome and penetrating stench. Finally there was tetanus, a terrible condition characterized by progressively intensifying convulsions and muscle seizures; tetanus was especially rampant among the newborn as well as in battlefield surgeries. Of those who survived the shock and pain of the surgery itself, more than half died from one of these infections. This was true even after surgical procedures that were relatively simple. As a result, surgery of any kind was usually a last resort.

Like other surgical procedures, cesarean sections were hopelessly dangerous and were usually performed only to save a fetus from a dead or dying mother.[10] The prohibitive dangers of cesarean section had one particularly grim consequence. In the major cities of Europe, most working-class children—perhaps 80 percent or more—were deficient in vitamin D; they nearly all suffered from rickets.[11] One early result of rickets is malformation of the pelvis. This usually meant that, when working-class girls became women, they were left with constricted birth canals; for them, vaginal delivery was long and difficult or even impossible. The medical literature contains many cases in which labor extended over several days or in which fetal limbs were torn from the body or the entire body was pulled away from the head in the course of delivery.[12] Sometimes, after days of labor, a dead fetus could be extracted only after it had been cut apart or its skull had been crushed. Such procedures were often fatal to the mother.

Surgery was usually performed in the same room and in the same bed to which the patient had been assigned. Thus, it often took place in large wards filled with other patients, most of whom were themselves either recovering from or awaiting surgery. This increased the opportunity for infection—and the suffering and screams of persons undergoing surgery vividly revealed what was in store for those whose turn had not yet come. In Vienna, partly as a humanitarian measure, the most terrible surgeries were performed in small rooms adjacent to the large surgical wards.[13]

While many medical beliefs and practices had remained almost the same for hundreds of years, there was one respect in which nineteenth-century medicine was changing. Physicians had become interested in the internal alterations associated with certain disease processes. This change in interest can be seen in the history of phthisis—a disease that was prevalent in that period.

In the eighteenth century, phthisis was a common disease. In some populations it accounted for about one-third of all adult deaths.[14] The first symptoms were persistent fever and cough; later, blood and pus were coughed up from the lungs. There was no effective treatment—victims gradually deteriorated until they died. Phthisis seemed especially common in Vienna, and physicians debated whether it was caused by dust from the busy streets or by the scandalous fast waltzes for which the city was becoming famous.

Until the late eighteenth century, there was little interest in understanding how fever and pus originated in the bodies of patients. The lungs and other internal organs of those who died from phthisis were seldom examined. In general, human cadavers were only rarely opened by physicians. When they were dissected, it was usually only to determine a cause of death or as an aid in the study of anatomy; no one seems to have been much interested in tracing disease symptoms to internal structural changes.

At about the beginning of the nineteenth century, studies by a series of French scientists—especially Gaspard-Laurent Bayle and René-Théophile-Hyacinthe Laennec—revealed that the symptoms of phthisis were associated with particular morbid alterations within the body. Because these internal changes could *explain* the symptoms, they seemed more fundamental than the symptoms themselves; and it appeared more precise and more enlightening to characterize phthisis in terms of the pathological changes, rather than in terms of the symptoms that physicians had long observed. Bayle and Laennec discovered that different internal alterations could cause the same symptoms. As a result, what had been thought of as a single disease—phthisis—was split into a variety of different diseases, depending on the internal changes that produced the symptoms.

Autopsies revealed that many cases of phthisis involved the formation of distinctive tumors or "tubers" in the lungs. Phthisis associated with tubers was distinguished from symptomatically similar cases in which the tubers were absent, and the tuberous disorder was thought of as a separate disease. In time, because the tubers were so characteristic, tuberous phthisis came to be known as tuberculosis.

Because the research in France shed so much light on phthisis and because phthisis was such a prominent disease, these studies became a model for research on other diseases. Physicians dissected corpses, sought morbid anatomical changes, and recharacterized familiar diseases in terms of the changes they were identifying. Such research was known as "pathological anatomy," and it gave physicians a whole new level of understanding: it seemed to provide a scientific basis for medicine. Not surprisingly, pathological anatomy became the main subject of medical research and became increasingly important in training new physicians.

Research and instruction in pathological anatomy depended on the availability of large numbers of human bodies, both diseased and dead. There were several reasons for this. First, to study any given disease, the investigators required access to many patients suffering from that disease. Only by examining many patients could researchers abstract from the peculiarities of individual patients and form a precise concept of the disease symptoms themselves. Second, internal pathological modifications could be identified and correlated with symptoms only by meticulously dissecting many corpses of persons who had died from each disease and by recording and comparing the results of such dissections. This was the only way of distinguishing normal post-mortem changes from the pathological changes that constituted the disease. Third, once a given disease process was understood, ever more patients and corpses were required to demonstrate these discoveries to successive generations of medical students. Fourth and finally, precise comprehension of pathological anatomy required more than lectures and demonstrations; everyone agreed that the subject could be mastered only through firsthand experience in the dissection of corpses, and this called for still more cadavers.

Thus, as pathological anatomy grew ever more central to medical thought, both research and training required access to ever larger numbers of disposable bodies, both living and dead. Where were these bodies to be found? And how could they be made available to the medical profession?

By the early nineteenth century, charity hospitals like the Viennese General Hospital were operating in most of the major cities of Europe. It seemed reasonable that persons treated in charity institutions should somehow repay society for the free care they received. It seemed especially equitable that this repayment should help advance and disseminate the medical skills from which the charity patients themselves were benefiting. The obvious solution was to use the charity patients as the raw material for medical research and training. Thus, persons admitted to gratis hospitals were expected to serve, as needed, in medical research and to submit themselves for use as teaching specimens in training new physicians. Moreover, it was understood that the hospitals retained control over the corpses of all the charity patients who died there. These corpses thereby became available for dissection by the medical personnel working in the institution.

During its first eighty-eight years of operation, 1.4 million patients were treated in Vienna's General Hospital. This number insured the continuous availability of patients suffering from virtually every common disease. Through these eighty-eight years, the hospital had a mortality rate of approximately 14 percent: about two hundred thousand patients died in the hospital.[15] The mortality rate was high in comparison with modern standards not only because medicine has become relatively more effective, but also because poor persons were regularly taken to the hospitals to die as a way of saving burial costs. The 14 percent mortality rate meant that, on average, the General Hospital morgue received about six new cadavers a day for every day of the year; all were available for dissection.

Thus, by collecting vast numbers of diseased and dying patients, the charity hospitals of Europe controlled precisely the resources deemed necessary for contemporary medical research and training.

Inevitably, the gratis hospitals became centers for the advancement and dissemination of medical knowledge. It is a profound historical coincidence that the interest of physicians was focused on pathological anatomy precisely as the charity hospitals were first making available a virtually unlimited supply of the resources on which that field depended.

Nineteenth-century medical research and training focused on two hospital institutions: the clinic and the morgue. Each clinic was assigned one or more rooms in a gratis hospital, and each such room contained from twenty to one hundred beds. These beds were occupied by patients selected from the general population of the hospital because they presented particularly enlightening cases of specific disorders. Each clinic was directed by a professor who conducted rounds, passing from bed to bed and discussing, in turn, the diseases exhibited by the different patients. The professor was followed by about thirty students. As the professor spoke, the students crowded around each bed, took turns examining the patient, and carefully recorded what they saw and heard. In this way the students learned to recognize the important diseases. This method of medical training, known as the "clinical system," originated in France at the end of the eighteenth century; it proved to be so effective that it was soon adopted throughout Europe.

In 1784 when Vienna's General Hospital began admitting patients, it included various divisions, concerned primarily with caring for the sick, and clinics, intended to train medical professionals. Each clinic specialized in a particular area of medicine depending on the interest of the professor who was in charge. When it opened, the Viennese General Hospital had three clinics, one each for internal medicine, surgery, and obstetrics. During the nineteenth century, more and more clinics were organized until, by the end of the century, there were nearly twenty. The new clinics studied particular kinds of disorders, and this fostered the emergence of medical specialties. Dermatology and ophthalmology were among the specialties that originated in the clinics of Vienna's General Hospital.

The other center for the study of medicine was the morgue. Here students correlated their clinic observations with internal morbid changes in corpses. Often, the same students who observed the symptoms of a given patient in the clinic would, within a few hours, dissect that patient's corpse in the morgue.

At Vienna's General Hospital, in each of the five years of study leading to a medical degree, students attended lectures both on ordinary gross anatomy and on pathological anatomy. Also as part of their training, students examined wax models, slightly larger than life, that displayed in amazing detail all the various organs and tissue systems of the body. Such models can be seen today in Vienna's medical history museum near the General Hospital. But firsthand dissections were far more enlightening than either lectures or the study of wax models, and medical students regularly spent several hours each day in the morgue dissecting cadavers. Indeed, in Vienna, the medical students spent so much time in the morgue that it became the customary gathering place where they met and passed time when they were not required to be elsewhere.[16] After working in the morgue, many students also carried parts of cadavers to their dwellings for further examination. One physician gave this advice to beginners:

> When you dissect, do not attack all the parts of the body at once. The best plan is to take the portion that you are examining to your room, and keep it fresh by plunging it into alcohol. Inspect it with care, and note down your observations. By these means, a head will occupy your time for five or six weeks very advantageously.[17]

The rise of pathological anatomy changed how physicians thought about disease. Earlier, individual diseases had been identified as particular collections of symptoms. The pathologists regarded symptoms as merely superficial manifestations of internal disease processes; whenever possible, they identified diseases as the morbid internal changes that caused the symptoms.

Joseph II, the enlightened Hapsburg innovator, died of phthisis in 1790, six years after the Viennese General Hospital began operation. The next few decades were an exceptionally turbulent period in Europe. In 1793 Joseph's sister, Marie Antoinette, was beheaded in Paris by French revolutionaries. A few years later, Napoleon gained control of France and used its army to force his own ideals on all of Europe. The Hapsburgs sent one army after another to fight the French, but their armies were usually defeated.

These developments completely extinguished the Hapsburgs' interest in innovation: in Austria, the Napoleonic era was a period of deepening conservatism. The Hapsburg monarch who presided over this period of defeat and retrenchment was Francis II, but he himself is remembered less vividly than is his opportunistic and reactionary prime minister, the notorious Clemens von Metternich. Metternich did everything he could to maintain the absolute powers of the Hapsburgs. As a result, he was hated and feared by reformers throughout the empire.

In Vienna, the general political conservatism of the period was reflected in doctrinal conservatism within the medical establishment. In 1806, Valentin von Hildenbrand was appointed professor of internal medicine at the General Hospital and within a few years became director of the entire institution. Hildenbrand championed the ancient notion that disease was caused by noxious atmospheric influences. He also believed that, at any given time, even the cases of different diseases shared a common essence that reflected existing atmospheric conditions. Acting on these beliefs, Hildenbrand observed and recorded various atmospheric factors such as temperature, pressure, relative humidity, and wind velocity. He also made precise records of the incidence of disease and death at the hospital and sought correlations between the weather conditions and the morbidity.

Because Hildenbrand believed that disease phenomena were mostly dependent on atmospheric factors, he was indifferent to what was happening within the bodies of his patients. However, the general European interest in pathological anatomy made it impossible to ignore the subject altogether, so Hildenbrand and the other physicians at the General Hospital conducted perfunctory autopsies. Under Hildenbrand, the Viennese lacked the confidence and dedication necessary to discover important correlations between case histories and autopsy results. Through the early years of the nineteenth century, the Austrians made only modest contributions to the rising field of pathological anatomy.

Hildenbrand's interest in the atmosphere also made him skeptical of active therapeutic intervention. Following the ancient Hippocratic tradition known as "expectant medicine," he believed that the best treatment was simply to allow patients to recover through their own natural healing processes. Consequently, in comparison to physicians in other European capitals, the Viennese were less aggressive in drawing blood and in administering other heroic therapies. The conservative inaction of Viennese physicians was frequently criticized by other European doctors and sometimes even by the citizens of Vienna, who expected their physicians to do more than merely watch them die.

After Hildenbrand's death in 1818, the physicians at the General Hospital grew progressively more interested in pathological anatomy. In 1821 the first full-time specialist in the field joined the hospital faculty. In 1833 Karl Rokitansky became the hospital's first full professor of pathological anatomy. Rokitansky, who is reputed to have personally dissected more than thirty thousand corpses over the course of his career, ultimately became one of the most important medical researchers ever associated with the Vienna medical school. His numerous careful dissections clearly revealed the correlations between disease symptoms and internal morbid alterations that earlier Viennese pathologists had sought but seldom found.

Rokitansky collected the strangest and most enlightening of his anatomical specimens and preserved them in large jars filled with alcohol. Today, Rokitansky's macabre collection of morbid anatomical remains—greatly amplified by the contributions of his successors—is open for public inspection at Vienna's General Hospital. It is now displayed in the Fools' Tower, the fantastic round tower built to house the insane. A tour of this museum and an inspection of its contents is not recommended for the fainthearted.

In the years following Rokitansky's appointment as professor of pathological anatomy, several other brilliant young researchers joined the faculty of the General Hospital. Jakob Kolletschka, who had been Rokitansky's student, specialized in forensic pathology. Ferdinand Hebra, the founder of modern dermatology, was the first physician at the General Hospital to specialize in skin diseases. But probably the most important of the young medical scientists at the General Hospital was the internist Josef Skoda. Skoda popularized the use of the stethoscope, which had been invented in France a generation earlier; he also developed percussion as a diagnostic technique. Percussion involved tapping the surfaces of the patient's body and classifying the resulting sounds. Before the discovery of X rays, this technique was the single most useful way of finding out what was happening within a living body. Skoda was able to associate the structural changes identified by Rokitansky with the sounds of percussion and with what he heard through his stethoscope. These associations enabled him to diagnose diseases with amazing speed and accuracy.

Rokitansky, Kolletschka, Hebra, and Skoda brought international fame to the medical school in Vienna. Partly because of their brilliant work and partly because Vienna's General Hospital provided an almost unlimited supply of diseased and dying patients, by the middle of the nineteenth century the hospital had become the world's foremost research and teaching institution. Physicians and advanced medical students from every part of the civilized world came there to study.

However, not everyone at the General Hospital was enthusiastic about the new work of Rokitansky and his disciples. Some senior faculty members remained faithful to Hildenbrand's view that atmospheric influences were more enlightening than morbid anatomical remains. Disagreement over this theoretical issue was exacerbated by other differences that were more emphatic, if less rational. First, there were the usual jealousies that are provoked on both sides when mediocre but firmly entrenched senior faculty members impede the aspirations of their more talented juniors. Second, there were sharply contrasting political sentiments. Most of the senior physicians were native Austrians and of Germanic extraction; by contrast, many of the brilliant younger physicians— including Skoda, Hebra, and Kolletschka—were from Bohemia or other parts of the Hapsburg empire. On the one hand, contemporary Viennese conservatism made native Austrians mistrust foreigners and their unorthodox ideas. On the other hand, rising nationalism made the Bohemians and Hungarians hostile to their Hapsburg masters and to the conservative native Austrians whom the Hapsburgs seemed invariably to favor. The inevitable result was a fierce power struggle within the Vienna medical school. In the 1840s, the Viennese medical faculty reflected, in miniature, the general nationalistic unrest that was about to convulse the Hapsburg empire as a whole.

Notes

1. Erna Lesky, *Meilensteine der Wiener Medizin* (Vienna: Wilhelm Maudrich, 1981), p. 42.

2. Lesky, p. 34.

3. Lesky, p. 34.

4. Lesky, p. 31.

5. "The Hospitals of Paris," *Lancet* 1 (1828–1829): 262–264.

6. Robert Thomas, *The Modern Practice of Physic*, 8th ed. (London: Longman, 1825), pp. 525 f.

7. "Syphilis Communicated by Leeches," *Lancet* 1 (1828–1829): 14.

8. K. Codell Carter, "On the Decline of Bloodletting in Nineteenth-Century Medicine," *Journal of Psychoanalytic Anthropology* 5 (1982): 219–234.

9. M. Delpech, "Case of a Wound of the Right Carotid Artery," *Lancet* 6 (1825): 210–213.

10. Edward Shorter, *A History of Women's Bodies* (London: Allen Lane, 1983), pp. 160 f.

11. Shorter, pp. 23–26.

12. George W. Balfour, "English and German Midwives," *Lancet* 2 (1855): 503.

13. Dieter Jetter, *Wien von den Anfängen bis um 1900*, vol. 5 of Geschichte des Hospitals (Wiesbaden, Germany: Franz Steiner, 1982), p. 51.

14. Robert Koch, "The Etiology of Tuberculosis," in *Essays of Robert Koch*, ed. and trans. K. Codell Carter (Westport, CT: Greenwood, 1987), p. 83.

15. Jetter, p. 28.

16. Gerster, "Das medicinische Wien," *Archiv für physiologische Heilkunde* 6 (1847): 320–329, 468–480, at p. 478.

17. Astley Cooper, "Surgical Lectures," *Lancet* 1 (1823): 1–9, at p. 5.

2

Childbed Fever

The maternity facilities of Vienna's General Hospital were located in the seventh courtyard on the east side of the institution. Originally, the maternity facilities included 178 beds, most of which were allocated to the obstetrical clinic and were available for charity patients. The clinic was responsible for training both obstetricians and midwives.

From 1798 until 1822, Johann Lukas Boer directed the Viennese maternity clinic. Boer's views on childbirth were compatible with Valentine von Hildenbrand's general therapeutic conservatism. Like Hildenbrand, Boer relied on nature rather than on aggressive medical intervention. Boer's attitude was reflected in his cautious use of forceps in delivery. Forceps, which had been invented at the beginning of the eighteenth century, became popular throughout Europe within a few decades. Although the use of metallic forceps increased the likelihood of damaging the tissues of delivering women, many physicians felt that the dangers were justified because forceps could reduce the time spent in labor. Some obstetricians used forceps in half of their deliveries; by contrast, of the nearly thirty thousand births that Boer supervised, forceps were used in just over one hundred cases.[1]

Boer did not draw blood from women who were about to deliver; and rather than administering the complex and dangerous drugs that were administered by many of his contemporaries, Boer prescribed nutritious foods, fresh air, and exercise. Hospital regulations required obstetrical students to practice on cadavers, but Boer ignored the regulations and allowed his students to use only fabricated leather models. He was also skeptical of pathological anatomy and did not routinely perform autopsies on women who died in his clinic.

After Hildenbrand died, Boer's disdain for pathological anatomy passed out of favor along with his other antiquated ideas and practices; in 1822 he was forced to resign. Boer was replaced by Johannes Klein, who had been Boer's student and assistant. Klein was an orthodox and unimaginative man. However, he was respected by his contemporaries and was deemed politically safe by the Viennese authorities. Klein immediately resumed the routine practice of performing autopsies, and—as stipulated by hospital regulations—he required his students to practice obstetrical manipulations on cadavers. One physician recorded that Klein's students regularly practiced using both female and fetal corpses so that training exercises would be as realistic as possible. He also observed that Vienna's General Hospital was probably the only facility in Europe with sufficient corpses to provide training of this kind.[2]

The original 178 beds in the maternity facility soon proved inadequate. In 1834, two new courtyards—referred to as the "eighth courtyard" and the "ninth courtyard"—were added to expand the maternity accommodations. The new buildings provided six hundred additional beds, most of which were in large rooms holding about thirty patients each. With this increase, the hospital could accommodate nearly eight hundred maternity patients—a figure approaching one-third of the total capacity of the entire hospital.

Since most of the new beds were filled by charity patients and were included within the obstetrical clinic, the clinic was too large to be supervised by a single professor, and it was divided into two sections of approximately equal size. The sections occupied adjacent rooms and shared some facilities. A second professor of obstetrics was appointed, and each of the two professors was allowed one assistant, who was normally appointed for a two-year term. While the professors conducted rounds, the assistants assumed responsibility for the daily care of patients and for teaching students both in the clinics and in the morgue.

Often, each obstetrical assistant would supervise twenty to thirty births within a twenty-four-hour period, and so it was necessary for them to be available at all times both day and night. For this reason, they were assigned small rooms within the clinic—rooms that served both as offices and as living space. Sixteen nurses were assigned to each section.[3] The nurses worked twenty-four-hour shifts; while on duty, they slept in the same rooms as their patients and, if necessary, in the same beds. As for the teaching function of the facility, the course in practical obstetrics lasted two months. In order that student obstetricians could attend all unusual deliveries, they too were provided accommodations within the clinic.[4]

Originally, half the male obstetrical students and half the female student midwives were assigned to each of the two sections of the clinic. However, in 1840 the students were separated as follows: all the males—normally between twenty and forty students— and about eight student midwives were assigned to one section, called the "first section." The remaining student midwives— about thirty in number—were assigned to the "second section."

Patients were assigned to the two sections as follows: all women who required special medical attention were placed in the first section—the section in which obstetricians were trained. Those not needing special attention were distributed between the two sections, depending on the day of the week on which they were admitted. Beginning at four o'clock on Monday afternoons, new arrivals were assigned to the first section. After twenty-four hours, beginning at four o'clock on Tuesday afternoons, new patients were placed in the second section. Admissions were changed daily in this way except that for forty-eight hours, from Friday afternoons through Sunday afternoons, all new patients were assigned to the first section. Thus, patients were admitted to the first section one day each week more than to the second. For this reason, and because the first section also received all the women with special medical problems, each year the first section admitted between four hundred and five hundred more patients than did the second.

In 1847 one physician gave this account of how deliveries were managed in the obstetricians' section:

> Four of the [eight] midwives are reserved for the night duty, and four for the day duty, and each of these must, in her turn, deliver a woman; but one is moreover called upon every eight days to act as the *Journalistin*, i.e., to watch and examine every case in labor admitted during a period of twenty-four hours. Two gentlemen (sometimes only one) are called upon to exercise, conjointly with the midwife in question, a similar function. In the discharge of this duty, they are allowed to repeat these [vaginal] examinations as frequently as they deem it necessary. But this is not all. When the membranes are ruptured, the midwife, according to order, is called to deliver the woman, and one gentleman . . . is also in attendance to witness the delivery. . . . These parties are allowed to make examinations, if they think fit. Again, the professor during his morning visit, and the assistant during the evening visit, not unfrequently make or allow examinations to be made by the gentlemen present, whenever a case of interest presents itself. Practically, therefore, every woman admitted must needs be examined by some five different persons at least, and this number may be doubled or even trebled. The practical instruction is also given in a private course, where the operations are performed upon the dead body of some female.[5]

The medical personnel who worked in the maternity clinics—students, nurses, and professors—all faced a constant risk of contracting syphilis. To appreciate the nature of the problem one must understand something about the disease.

Syphilis can occur in different forms. Ordinarily, within a few weeks of being infected, victims experience a small open sore at the infection site. However, in some cases there is no open wound at all. Even if there is an open sore, it may cause little discomfort and resemble other minor skin infections; so it is easy to overlook. The primary ulceration may gradually heal, and several weeks may pass without symptoms. Next, the victim may develop a rash; at the same time, rough open sores may form within the mouth or on the membranes inside the genitals. However, these symptoms may also be mild and resemble the symptoms of other diseases. Syphilis is most contagious during these early stages. Body fluids or discharges from the open and moist sores on the skin or within the mouth or genitals usually contain vast numbers of syphilis organisms. If these organisms are introduced into surface wounds elsewhere on the body or on other victims, they readily form new lesions.

In time, all the symptoms of syphilis may disappear spontaneously, and the disease may enter a latent phase. Twenty years or more may pass without symptoms; in the latent period, syphilis is not ordinarily contagious. However, even in the absence of overt symptoms, the causal organisms may be attacking various tissues inside the body, including the central nervous system. Finally the disease may show itself again, in a third or tertiary stage. The victim develops new symptoms depending on which tissues have been destroyed by the syphilis organisms; these symptoms may arise slowly over a space of several months. If the central nervous system has been attacked, there may be minor changes in personality as well as headaches and insomnia. The victim may suffer memory loss and become irritable. Often there is a loss of judgment, and the victim becomes indifferent to the affairs of ordinary life. These changes may occur so gradually that even friends and family members do not realize what is happening. As the disease grows worse, victims may suffer a form of paralysis that begins with the development of a characteristic slapping gait and gradually spreads to other parts of the body. In time, victims may be unable to walk or stand; they may become bedridden and unable even to feed themselves.

Syphilis was common in nineteenth-century Europe. Most of the women who delivered in gratis maternity clinics were unmarried, and many supplemented their meager incomes by working as prostitutes. At any given time, several of the women in the clinics would have been syphilitic. There being no effective diagnostic tests, it was impossible to be sure exactly who had the disease. Syphilis was known to be contagious; but otherwise, little was understood about how it spread or how it could be prevented. There were no standard prophylactic measures such as the use of surgical gloves. Since persons associated with the clinic performed dozens of vaginal examinations each day, they were regularly exposed. Medical personnel with minor cuts or abrasions were especially at risk. Many contracted syphilis while conducting routine examinations; but because the disease often has no distinctive symptoms in its early stages, these clinic personnel may never have known when or how they became infected. Often, the first unmistakable signs did not appear until twenty years after infection.

Primary and secondary syphilis were generally treated by administering nearly lethal doses of mercury, but everyone recognized that even this treatment was ineffective once the disease reached the tertiary stage. There was no effective treatment and the outcome was certain. Obstetricians joked grimly about the disease, and many regarded it as an almost inevitable consequence of their years of work in the maternity clinics.

Various procedures at Vienna's maternity facilities reflected the humanitarian goals of the institution. To ensure the confidentiality and privacy of patients, admission was conducted within the maternity facility itself rather than through the general administrative offices of the hospital. No visitors—not even regular hospital physicians or staff—were allowed in the paying maternity wards, and access to the entire facility was strictly controlled.

At admission, each charity patient was required to write her name and address on a sheet of paper that was then folded, sealed, and placed on a shelf by her bed. If a patient died, the paper was opened so that her family or neighbors could be notified; if she lived, the unopened paper was returned to her when she was discharged. Otherwise, maternity patients were not required to disclose their names or any other personal information to anyone. Maternity patients were even allowed to wear masks during their entire stay, so that neither the hospital staff nor other patients could later identify them.

In order to reduce the likelihood of abortions—and because it was useful to have available teaching specimens from all stages of pregnancy—women were accepted into the maternity clinic at any time during pregnancy and were allowed to remain there as long as they cared to do so, without charge, even after giving birth. Since the clinic provided better food and lodging than many indigent women could provide for themselves, some women spent three months or longer in the hospital. In return, beyond the usual requirements of being available for use in medical research and teaching, patients were expected to perform housekeeping tasks in the clinic, to sew and knit clothing for the poor, and to nurse orphaned babies.

Associated with the maternity clinic was a foundlings home for the newborn babies of charity patients. Clinic policy—intended to encourage women to deliver in the clinic and, therefore, to be available for use as teaching specimens—specified that infants delivered outside the hospital would be accepted in the foundlings home only in return for the payment of a fee. However, those born suddenly and unexpectedly to women who had actually been on their way to the hospital were accepted gratis as though they had been delivered in the clinic itself.

Like the charity maternity clinics of the period, the foundlings homes were a consequence of humanitarian ideals, but they fell short of expectations. In the Viennese facility—as in similar institutions throughout Europe—only a few babies survived even one year. Many died from congenital syphilis, but most died in the terrible gastro-intestinal epidemics that periodically swept the institutions, killing virtually all the otherwise healthy inmates. One British physician who visited the Viennese foundlings home observed that each child

> was provided with a comforter consisting of a piece of linen stuffed with bread and milk. The food in this was supposed to be changed every twenty-four hours, but human nature being what it is, in many cases it was only renewed after many days. This piece of fermenting filth was stuffed into the child's mouth at every opportunity. Hot one minute, cold the next, and always saturated with saliva, no wonder it was a most efficient means of propagating disease.[6]

In the seventy years between 1784 and 1854, of the 293,544 babies accepted into the Viennese foundlings home, 228,818— almost 80 percent—died before they were adopted or became old enough to be discharged.[7]

In an attempt to reduce this horrible loss, Joseph II ordered that every healthy baby be removed from the foundlings home and consigned to a private family as soon after birth as possible. The family received a state subsidy in exchange for raising the infant. This program had little impact on mortality, but for a time it was popular among Austrian farmers: the law required each farm family to provide one conscript for the Hapsburg armies; accepting a child from the foundlings home promised to provide not only subsidized farm labor but also a relatively painless way of meeting the military conscription. Because of this practice, contemporaries joked that the Hapsburgs defended themselves with an army of bastards.

Hospitals like Vienna's were intended to provide safe and humane facilities in which indigent women could give birth and, in many respects, were indeed a great improvement over earlier institutions. But women who delivered in the clinics were much more likely to die in childbirth than women who delivered elsewhere, and the clinics soon gained a sinister reputation among the very women they were intended to serve. In the clinics, women were especially vulnerable to a particularly horrible disease known as "childbed fever" or "puerperal fever" (from the word *puerpera*, meaning a woman who had just given birth).

One eighteenth-century English physician described childbed fever as follows:

> The disease . . . is ushered in, from the second to the fourth day of confinement, by shivering, accompanied by acute pain radiating from the region of the uterus, increased on pressure, and gradually extending all over the abdomen, with suppression of lochia and milk, much accelerated pulse, furred tongue, great heat of skin, and a peculiar pain in the sinciput [forehead]. [Patients usually have] short breathing, their knees drawn up, and great anxiety of countenance.[8]

Once the symptoms were established, puerperal fever was fatal in more than half of all cases.

Medical literature from the eighteenth and early nineteenth centuries contains hundreds of case histories of victims of childbed fever. Here is a typical account:

> Mrs. Y_____, a lady near the Abbey in Westminster, young, and of a strong and healthy habit, after a labour perfectly natural, was suddenly attacked with a violent shivering fit, the third day after delivery, being the 1st of January 1770.

She was also affected with a thrilling, uncommon sensation, as if a cold, wet sheet had been applied round her body.

She complained of headache, and was sick at stomach; during the excess of febrile heat, her pulse beat 130 times in a minute, and was more full and strong than usual in this fever; her countenance was florid, and much altered from its natural state, having an unusual stare with her eyes.

Small portions of emetic tartar [antimony] . . . were given with the saline mixture every four hours. She diluted plentifully with barley-water and balm-tea, but did not perspire.

The second day after the attack a violent bilious purging came on; the antimonial powders were then given by longer intervals, . . .

The fever and diarrhoea continued very violent for three or four days; her belly swelled, and she frequently complained of much pain at the bottom of her stomach, and towards the navel. Sometimes there seemed to be obscure signs of a remission in the morning; but towards the evening the fever again returned with violence. [The physician records that he drew eight ounces of blood and administered various medications.] . . .

A few days before her death she was delirious; her eyes were bloodshot and filled with involuntary tears; at the same time a miliary eruption appeared very thick on her breast and body, and her stools, which were frequent and very fetid, came away insensibly.

Leeches were then applied to her temples; the clysters [enemas] were repeated, and her strength was supported by nourishment and wine; but all without salutary effect, for on the 12th of January she died, and several hours before her death became perfectly sensible.[9]

Healthy young women concluding their first pregnancies seemed especially vulnerable to this horrible disease.

Accounts of isolated cases of what may have been childbed fever appear in Greek and Roman medical texts. However, the earliest recorded epidemic occurred in the Hôtel-Dieu of Paris in 1664. According to the published account, newly delivered women began dying in large numbers. Physicians opened the cadavers of some of the women and found them full of abscesses. A careful search for the cause revealed that the delivery room was located immediately above a room for wounded patients. The physicians concluded that

> coarse and infectious vapors, which arose from the wounds and ulcers of the injured bodies, created a mass of impure and malignant air. This air perpetually rose upward and was inhaled day and night by the newly delivered women. The women fell into a bloody flux that ended only with their death.[10]

Physicians noticed that the number of fever victims corresponded directly to the number of patients in the lower room and to the relative humidity of the atmosphere.

Through the following two centuries, similar epidemics were described with increasing frequency. By the middle of the eighteenth century, the disease had become common enough to be given the specific names by which it is still known. Over the next hundred years, epidemics of childbed fever continued to devastate the large maternity clinics of Europe.

In the eighteenth century, women in the clinics during epidemic years were at significantly greater risk than those who delivered at home. Otherwise, the risk in the clinics was probably about the same as elsewhere.[11] However, by the middle of the nineteenth century, mortality in the clinics had increased substantially. In 1875 one physician estimated that, through the early and middle decades of the century, about 1 in 29 women who delivered in the clinics died, while only about 1 in 212 of those who delivered at home died.[12] Modern historians arrive at similar estimates.[13]

There was considerable variation in morbidity among the hospitals themselves and from one year to another. Over intervals of several weeks, some smaller hospitals reported mortality rates of nearly 100 percent. The Maternité in Paris probably had the highest sustained mortality of any large institution: between 1861 and 1864, almost one-fifth of all deliveries resulted in the death of the mother.[14]

While Boer supervised the obstetrical clinic in Vienna, the mortality rate for childbed fever averaged about 1 percent—a very favorable rate. Under Klein, there were two important changes. First, total mortality rose immediately, increasing to about 5 percent. But the incidence of the disease was increasing throughout Europe, and even at 5 percent, the patients in Vienna were safer than those in many other institutions. Thus, in spite of the astounding increase in mortality, childbed fever was not regarded as a problem unique to, or unusually troublesome in, Vienna. However, because so many women delivered in the Viennese hospital, even its relatively low mortality rate involved hundreds of deaths each year. Second, before 1840, the two sections of the maternity clinic had approximately equal mortality rates; beginning in 1840, when the male obstetrical students were all assigned to the first section and most of the female student midwives were assigned to the second section, mortality in the first section was consistently four or five times greater than in the second. Indeed, while the mortality in the second section was seldom above 2 percent, in the first section it was often 10 percent or more.

It soon became obvious that the first section was more dangerous than the second, but no one was exactly sure why. One common explanation was this: since more women were admitted to the first section each year than to the second section, the first section must be more crowded. Physicians believed that the air in crowded hospitals became contaminated by dangerous vapors called "miasms." Thus, it seemed logical that the miasms would be more intense and therefore more lethal in the crowded first section of the maternity clinic than in the second. But little was done to address the problem, and the measures taken had little effect.

The official mortality records at the maternity clinic were strictly confidential. But because there were so many deaths, it was common knowledge that maternity patients were in danger there, and that the first section—the section with the male students— was considerably more dangerous than the second. Local women dreaded the prospect of going to the clinic to give birth.

To reduce their chances of contracting childbed fever, while still qualifying for free postpartum care and the services of the foundlings home, some women in labor simply wandered the streets of Vienna until they gave birth—usually in a doorway or in the empty fields just outside the old city walls. Then, carrying their babies in their arms, they walked to the hospital and applied for admission. Since they had delivered while on their way to the hospital, they and their babies were accepted without charge and received the same benefits as were provided to women who had delivered in the clinic. Giving birth even under such horrible circumstances was safer than doing so in the clinic. In discussing this practice, one contemporary obstetrician pointed out that as many as one hundred patients a month were admitted after having delivered on their way to the hospital.[15] Many— perhaps most—of these women had intentionally delayed arrival and had given birth on the street rather than risk delivering in the clinic.

Physicians and public authorities were aware of the ravages of childbed fever: even in official documents the maternity clinics were referred to as ''death traps'' or ''houses of death.''[16] The governments of Europe initiated inquiries, and the disease received extensive attention in medical texts. There were intensive efforts to identify the causes of the disease. But, not surprisingly, physicians reported only the same general causes that they found for all other diseases.

In 1773 a prominent British obstetrician observed that childbed fever could be caused when the "tightness of stays and petticoat bindings, and the weight of the pockets and of the petticoats" press the intestines and block excretion thereby forcing the body to reabsorb its own wastes. Other causes were said to include a sedentary inactive life, improper diet, the attendance of friends in a small room, a large fire, air "rendered foul and unfit for respiration," strong liquors mixed with warm waters, too many coverings, stagnation of lochia in the womb, damp and close houses, want of cleanliness, the ascension of miasms from families living below, or hospital miasms. The physician complained that "the breasts, if drawn at all, are not drawn until several days after delivery, when they are so full as to be perfectly gorged, and as hard as stones, by which means the first milk . . . is thrown back into the circulation," thus leading to milk fever and to childbed fever. He observed that the disease could be caused through "violence by instruments or by the hands in delivery."[17]

A contemporary German physician ascribed the disease to rough treatment, retention or suppression of menstruation, chilling, cold drinks, depressing passions, the inhabitation of damp or wet dwellings and suppression of the breast or abdominal-genital secretions. He observed that, once childbed fever began, it could spread by contagion. He warned that it could be conveyed by secretions—especially genital secretions—from ill individuals and that a contagium could be generated when many patients were crowded together without adequate ventilation. He warned against sharing bathtubs, lavatories, and underwear.[18]

One British physician observed that, in different cases, childbed fever had been traced

> to difficult labour; to inflammation of the uterus; to accumulation of noxious humours, set in motion by labour; to violent mental emotion, stimulants, and obstructed perspiration; to miasmata, admission of cold air to the body, and into the

uterus; to hurried circulation; to suppression of lacteal secretion; diarrhea; liability to putrid contagion from changes in the humours during pregnancy; hasty separation of the placenta; binding the abdomen too tight; sedentary employment; stimulating or spare diet; [or to] fashionable dissipation.[19]

Because childbed fever was sometimes attributed to local miasms, when an epidemic became especially intense in a given maternity clinic, the clinic was generally closed, the walls scrubbed and painted, and new linen and bedding procured. But none of these measures was reliable; often the first patients admitted after such efforts would die from the disease. One physician suggested trying to control local miasms by putting basins of chlorinated calcium between the patients' beds.

Therapy for childbed fever usually involved bloodletting. Blood was taken both locally by applying leeches and generally by opening veins or arteries. In 1848 a British physician described his approach:

I immediately order eight or a dozen leeches to be scattered over the abdomen, and to be followed by a linseed or bran poultice; the vagina to be washed out with tepid water, and, if the lochia be fetid, an injection of chloride of soda used; large doses of calomel [mercury] and opium to be given every three hours, and beef-tea administered at intervals; the calomel to be pushed to approaching ptyalism [poisoning]: when this commences, the calomel to be remitted. Should the pain not yield quickly under these means, I either apply more leeches, or, if the strength will not allow of them, make use of the turpentine poultice; the effect of this last is in many cases almost magical.[20]

A few years later, an American physician recommended this treatment:

> Let it be carefully treasured in memory, that there is no
> specific [remedy] for this disease . . . [but that] the prompt
> abstraction of blood is called for; take from the arm from
> twelve to thirty ounces of blood [one to three pints], depend-
> ing, of course, on the urgency of the case, and in order that
> there may be nothing equivocal in the impression made on
> the system, bleed from a large orifice, let there be a bold
> and full stream; in one word, make your patient faint;
> syncope [fainting] will more readily be accomplished by
> placing the patient in the sitting position during the abstrac-
> tion of blood. . . . The next indication will be a free action
> on the bowels. . . . We have an important adjuvant in
> blisters, after the intensity of the disease is somewhat broken;
> instead, however, of placing them on the abdomen, I greatly
> prefer applying them on the internal surface of the thighs,
> immediately over the femoral arteries.[21]

The practice in Vienna was similar. In the 1820s, one physician
gave this account:

> They employed in most cases, immediately on the commence-
> ment of the disease, repeated venesection [opening of the
> veins], the application of leeches, emollient cataplasms
> [medicated substances spread over the skin], emollient
> clysters [enemas]; at a later period, blisters, with the cor-
> responding internal remedies; in some cases calomel and
> other celebrated remedies; and in some, where gastric affec-
> tions at first predominated, emetics [to induce vomiting].[22]

Twenty years later, in the 1840s, treatment had not changed
significantly. One contemporary recorded that therapy at Vienna's
General Hospital usually involved massive local and general
measures intended to remove heat from the body—especially
bloodletting.[23] Another physician recorded that corpses from the
Viennese maternity clinic usually arrived in the morgue with
enormous open sores on the interiors of the thighs from the

blistering agents that had been applied in attempting to remove poisons from the body.[24]

Following the program of pathological anatomy, physicians tried to understand childbed fever by studying the morbid changes they found within its victims. Pathologists gave particular attention to changes in the uterus. This seemed reasonable since the disease was associated with birth and since autopsies often disclosed pathological changes in that organ. However, childbed fever left different and apparently unrelated morbid remains that did not always involve the uterus. According to the principles of pathological anatomy, this meant that childbed fever was not a single disease, but a group of symptomatically related diseases; and some physicians stopped talking about childbed fever and fell back on terms like "endometritis" (inflammation of the mucous membrane of the uterus), "metrophlebitis" (inflammation of the veins of the uterus), "meningitis" (inflammation of the tissues surrounding the brain and spinal cord), or "peritonitis" (inflammation of the serous membrane lining the walls of the abdomen). This way of thinking seemed more precise; but when it came to treatment, it led only to the same ineffective results.

The time had come for someone to look at the facts and see something quite different. That person, Ignaz Semmelweis, became Johannes Klein's assistant in the first section of Vienna's maternity clinic in 1846.

Notes

1. Erna Lesky, *The Vienna Medical School of the Nineteenth Century* (Baltimore: Johns Hopkins, 1976), p. 53.

2. Gerster, "Das medicinische Wien," *Archiv für physiologische Heilkunde* 6 (1847): 320–329, 468–480, at p. 476.

3. C. H. F. Routh, "On the Causes of the Endemic Puerperal Fever of Vienna," *Medico-chirurgical Transactions* 32 (1849): 27–40, at p. 28.

4. Gerster, p. 475.

5. Routh, pp. 28 f.

6. T. G. Wilson, *Victorian Doctor: Being the Life of Sir William Wilde* (London: Methuen, 1942), pp. 109 f.

7. Erna Lesky, *Meilensteine der Wiener Medizin* (Vienna: Wilhelm Maudrich, 1981), p. 38.

8. C. M. Miller, "On the Treatment of Puerperal Fever," *Lancet* 2 (1848): 262.

9. John Leake, *Practicle Observations on the Child-bed Fever* (1772; reprint in Fleetwood Churchill, ed., *Essays on the Puerperal Fever* [London: Sydenham Society, 1849]), pp. 180 f.

10. Quoted in Sophia Jex-Blake, "Puerperal Fever: An Inquiry into Its Nature and Treatment," M.D. diss., University of Bern, 1877, p. 1.

11. Margaret DeLacy, "Puerperal Fever in Eighteenth-Century Britain," *Bulletin of the History of Medicine* 63 (1989): 521–556, at pp. 544 f.

12. L. Landau, "Das Puerperalfieber und die Gebärhäuser," *Berliner klinische Wochenschrift* 12 (1875): 150–152, 166–169, at p. 151.

13. DeLacy, p. 538.

14. DeLacy, p. 538.

15. Ignaz Semmelweis, *The Etiology, Concept, and Prophylaxis of Childbed Fever*, ed. and trans. K. Codell Carter (Madison: University of Wisconsin, 1983), pp. 80 f.

16. Semmelweis, pp. 110, 200, 215.

17. Charles White, *A Treatise on the Management of Pregnant and Lying-in Women* (London: E. and C. Dilly, 1773), pp. 2–11.

18. Lucas Schönlein, *Allgemeine und Specielle Pathologie und Therapie* (St. Gallen, Switzerland: Litteratur-Comptoir, 1841), pp. 266 f., 284–289, 325.

19. J. M. Waddy, "On Puerperal Fever," *Lancet* 2 (1845): 671 f.

20. Miller, p. 262.

21. G. S. Bedford, *The Principles and Practice of Obstetrics*, 4th ed. (New York: William Wood, 1868), p. 183.

22. "Documents Relative to the History of the Malignant Puerperal Fever Which Prevailed in the Lying-in Institution in Vienna, from the Beginning of August to the middle of November 1819," *Edinburgh Medical and Surgical Journal* 22 (1824): 83–91, at p. 88.

23. Gerster, p. 477.

24. Wilson, pp. 107 f.

3

Semmelweis's Discovery

After rising in the Black Forest, the Danube river flows a thousand miles eastward to the Black Sea. Near the middle of its journey it leaves its eastward course and flows two hundred miles almost due south, bisecting the fertile plains of modern-day Hungary.

About eleven hundred years ago, in the spring of the year 895, Magyar tribes invaded these plains from the east and assimilated or encompassed the small bands of Slavs, Avars, and Franks already living there. Thus began the Hungarian nation. In time, the Magyars accepted Christianity and became part of the loose feudal organization known as the Holy Roman Empire. Being on the eastern edge of the empire, Hungary was particularly vulnerable to incursions by nomadic tribes and by other non-European powers.

By the fifteenth century, the Ottoman Turks—advancing northwest through the Balkans—were attacking Hungary's southern border. In 1526, after a century of intermittent warfare, the Hungarians were decisively defeated at the battle of Mohacs, and the Turks occupied central Hungary. Only the eastern and western edges of the country—known respectively as ''Transylvania'' and ''Royal Hungary''—remained relatively independent from the Turks. Transylvania is now part of Romania, and Royal Hungary has been annexed to Austria as the province of Burgenland. Modern-day Hungary is approximately that part of the ancient realm conquered by the Turks.

Near the end of the seventeenth century—after about 150 years of Turkish occupation—a combined European army dislodged the Turks and drove them back to the south. The Austrian Hapsburgs, as Holy Roman emperors, had been nominal kings of Hungary and liege lords of the Hungarian nobility since long before the Turkish occupation. As the Turkish threat was dispelled, the Hapsburgs reestablished and intensified their dominion over Hungary. Hungary passed from Turkish to Hapsburg rule.

The Hapsburg empire consisted of dozens of ethnically and linguistically distinct nationalities that occupied central Europe and the Balkans. To increase efficiency and to reinforce their own control, the Hapsburgs appointed mostly Germanic clergy, generals, and administrators. The Hapsburgs also rewarded the loyal nobility by giving or selling them enormous tracts of land in various parts of the empire. Thus, much of Hungary was directly owned or otherwise administered by Germanic nobles, most of whom lived in Vienna. The Hungarians and the other non-Germanic populations in the empire felt oppressed and exploited by their Austrian rulers and administrators. By the beginning of the nineteenth century, the Hapsburgs remained in control, but they faced periodic insurrections and rising nationalism in Hungary as in other parts of their empire.

Budapest, the capital of Hungary, is located on the banks of the south-flowing Danube about seventy miles east of Vienna. Modern Budapest is the union of several previously independent communities that gradually merged. The two largest of these communities were Buda, which grew up around medieval fortifications located on the hilly west bank of the Danube, and Pest, a commercial city on the flat east bank. In the early nineteenth century, the various communities that were merging into Budapest had a combined population of about seventy-five thousand; thus, the Hungarian city had approximately one-third the population of Vienna. Budapest was inhabited by a mixture of different ethnic groups, the most populous of which were the Magyars, Germans, Slavs, and Serbs.

Just below the south end of the Buda castle—facing the Danube and encircled on three sides by steep hills—is a flat area known as Tabán. At present, Tabán contains an eighteenth-century baroque church, a few apartment buildings, and a modern traffic interchange surrounded by nondescript grassy parks; it is a sleepy and relatively uninteresting section of modern Budapest. However, in the nineteenth century, Tabán was an independent community and an active center of commerce. For a time it was the western end of an important boat bridge that spanned the Danube, and the area was filled with busy shops and markets.

At the beginning of the nineteenth century, József Semmelweis was a prominent grocer in Tabán. Before moving to Tabán in about 1800, Semmelweis had lived in the western part of Hungary—in the narrow strip that remained just outside Turkish control and that is now part of Austria. The Semmelweis family probably descended from a tribe of Franks that inhabited western Hungary even before the Magyars invaded in the tenth century. Semmelweis's grocery store, which was called "To the White Elephant," was located on the ground floor at one end of a long two-story building decorated in the baroque style.

In 1810, at the age of thirty-two, József Semmelweis married Terézia Müller, the daughter of a prosperous coachwright who had migrated to Budapest from Bavaria. József and Terézia Semmelweis lived in an apartment on the second floor of the same building in which József's store was located. Ten children were born to the couple; all were baptized in the Tabán church about one hundred yards from the house in which they lived.

Like many other middle-class commercial families living in Budapest, the Semmelweis family spoke a Germanic dialect, but the children learned Hungarian in school and spoke it fluently. On school registration forms, the Semmelweis children consistently identified themselves as Hungarian, although they were of Germanic extraction. Ignaz Semmelweis, the fifth child in the family, was born 1 July 1818.

The building in which the Semmelweis family lived and worked still stands on Apród Street in Tabán. The rooms in which they lived are now a museum for the history of medicine. Many of the museum exhibits deal with the life and work of Ignaz Semmelweis. Some books, furniture, and personal effects that belonged to Semmelweis during his lifetime are also displayed.

We have only a few hints about Ignaz Semmelweis's personality. The diary of one contemporary, now lost, is reported to have described him as "of a happy disposition, truthful and open-minded, extremely popular with friends and colleagues."[1] His writings suggest that he was energetic, impulsive, thorough, and sensitive. He described himself as one who disliked and shunned all controversy. A few years after Semmelweis died, one Viennese colleague (in an obituary notice for a different physician) referred to him as "the genial Semmelweis."[2]

After completing his primary and secondary education mostly in parochial schools in Budapest, in the autumn of 1837 Ignaz Semmelweis entered the University of Vienna. Semmelweis began studying law; but in the following year, for reasons that are no longer known, he changed to medicine. He completed an M.D. in 1844.

Semmelweis applied for the position of assistant in Josef Skoda's clinic for internal medicine, but another physician was chosen instead. Semmelweis then decided to specialize in obstetrics. He twice completed the two-month obstetrics course in the first section of the Viennese General Hospital's maternity clinic. The course was taught by Johannes Klein's son-in-law, Baptist Johann Chiari. Semmelweis was awarded a master's degree in midwifery.

On 1 July 1846, his twenty-eighth birthday, Semmelweis was appointed Klein's assistant in the first section of the Viennese maternity clinic. As assistant, Semmelweis was expected to examine the patients each morning in preparation for Klein's rounds, to assist Klein with obstetrical operations, to supervise difficult deliveries, and to teach the obstetrical students both by conducting demonstrative autopsies in the morgue and by leading afternoon rounds in the clinic. He was also responsible for the clerical records of his section.

In the first section of the maternity clinic, Semmelweis was immediately confronted by the horrible reality of childbed fever. Because it was commonly known that the first section had a much higher mortality rate than the second, women tried to avoid being assigned there. Semmelweis tells us that he was frequently obliged to "witness moving scenes in which patients, kneeling and wringing their hands, beg to be released in order to seek admission to the second section."[3] He also writes that "the disrespect displayed by the [hospital] employees toward the personnel of the first section made me so miserable that life seemed worthless."[4] Despite his best efforts, the incidence of childbed fever in the first section actually increased after he became assistant. As Semmelweis himself tells us, he was bewildered and tormented by the high mortality rate in his section.

In keeping with his training in pathological anatomy, Semmelweis tried to understand puerperal fever by dissecting its victims. He obtained permission from Karl Rokitansky to examine the corpses of all the women who died in the clinic. Semmelweis performed these autopsies early each morning before beginning his regular duties in the first section, and he tells us he was particularly diligent in carrying out this loathsome task. However, he found only a confusing variety of morbid alterations—nothing that explained the difference in mortality rates between the two sections.

The first and second sections of the maternity clinic were adjacent and even shared some facilities. From their proximity,

Semmelweis concluded that any atmospheric influences would necessarily be the same in both clinics and, therefore, such influences could not account for the difference in mortality. The only possibility was that the increased morbidity in the first section was caused by something within the section itself.

In an essay published one year before Semmelweis became Klein's assistant, Eduard Lumpe had endorsed the popular view that most cases of childbed fever in Vienna's clinic were caused by harmful miasms generated within the clinic itself. Because the first section admitted more patients than the second, Lumpe inferred that the first section must be overcrowded, and he further concluded that the harmful miasms were not dispelled from the first section as readily as from the second. According to Lumpe, this was the only possible explanation for the difference in mortality between the sections. Semmelweis quickly saw that Lumpe's explanation was inadequate.

> If overcrowding were the cause of death, mortality in the second section would have been larger because the second section was more crowded than the first. Because of the bad reputation of the first section, everyone sought admission to the second. For this reason, the second section was often unable to resume admissions at the specified time as it was impossible to accommodate new arrivals. Or if the second section began to admit, within a few hours it was necessary to resume admitting patients to the first section because the passageway was crowded with such a great number of persons awaiting admission to the second section. In a short time all the free places were taken. In the five years I was associated with the first section, not once did overcrowding make it necessary to reopen admission to the second section.[5]

Semmelweis acknowledged that there were more births in the first section than in the second; but, he observed, for that very reason the first section had been assigned more beds than the second.

In terms of the percentage of occupied beds, the first section was actually the less crowded of the two.

Semmelweis also became persuaded that none of the other recognized causes of childbed fever could account for the difference in mortality. He considered all the usual factors such as inadequate ventilation, too much blood in the circulation, disturbances caused by the pregnant uterus, stagnation of the circulation, decreased weight caused by the emptying of the uterus; protracted labor, wounding of the inner surface of the uterus in delivery, imperfect contractions, faulty involutions of the uterus during maternity, the volume of secreted milk, and the death of the fetus. But because of the way in which patients were assigned to the two sections, the women in the second section were equally vulnerable to all these factors; hence, none of these conditions could explain the difference in mortality.

> The high mortality was also attributed to the section's practice of admitting only single women in desperate circumstances. These women had been obliged throughout their pregnancies to support themselves by hard work. They were miserable and in great need, often malnourished, and many had attempted to induce miscarriages. But if these conditions constituted the cause, the mortality rate in the second section should have been the same, since the same type of women were admitted there.[6]

Being unable to explain the difference in mortality by any of the recognized etiological factors, Semmelweis began trying to eliminate every difference between the two sections, however harmless it may have appeared. He determined that the same laundry contractor cleaned the linen for both sections and that the same food was served to all the patients.

> The reader can appreciate my perplexity . . . when I, like a drowning person grasping straws, discontinued supine

deliveries, which had been customary in the first section, in favor of deliveries from a lateral position. I did this for no other reason than that the latter were customary in the second section. I did not believe that the supine position was so detrimental that additional deaths could be attributed to its use. But in the second section deliveries were performed from a lateral position and the patients were healthier. Consequently, we also delivered from the lateral position, so that everything would be exactly as in the second section.[7]

Semmelweis even considered the religious practices of the two sections.

The hospital chapel was so located that when the priest was summoned to administer last rites in the second section he could go directly to the room set aside for ill patients. On the other hand, when he was summoned to the first section he had to pass through five other rooms because the room containing ill patients was sixth in line from the chapel. According to accepted Catholic practice, when visiting the sick to administer last rites, the priest generally arrived in ornate vestments and was preceded by a sacristan who rang a bell. This was supposed to occur only once in twenty-four hours. Yet twenty-four hours is a long time for someone suffering from childbed fever. Many who appeared tolerably healthy at the time of the priest's visit, and who therefore did not require last rites, were so ill a few hours later that the priest had to be summoned again. One can imagine the impression that was created on the other patients when the priest came several times a day, each time accompanied by the clearly audible bell. Even to me it was very demoralizing to hear the bell hurry past my door. I groaned within for the victim who had fallen to an unknown cause. The bell was a painful admonition to seek this unknown cause with all my powers. It had been proposed that even this difference in the two sections explained the different mortality rates. . . .

I appealed to the compassion of the servant of God and arranged for him to come by a less direct route, without bells, and without passing through the other rooms. Thus, no one outside the room containing the ill patients knew of the priest's presence.[8]

The two sections were made identical in every possible respect, but no reduction in the high mortality rate of the first section occurred.

The assistants in the various clinics in Vienna's General Hospital were normally appointed for two years. However, in November 1846, after only four months as Klein's assistant, Semmelweis was required to withdraw because his predecessor, Franz Breit, found it necessary to return to his post in the clinic. In the same month that Breit returned, officials at the hospital conjectured that the presence of large numbers of male students in the first section could contribute to the high mortality. Only married women who had themselves given birth were accepted as student midwives. Some authorities speculated that such women were more gentle in conducting examinations than were the unmarried male students; perhaps this had something to do with the morbidity. Consequently, the number of males accepted into the obstetrical course was reduced from forty-two to twenty, and the number of foreign students who were admitted was limited to two. Remarkably enough, the mortality rate in the first section immediately dropped, and there was some optimism that a solution had been found.

During the winter of 1846, while Breit supervised the first section, Semmelweis studied English with the intention of traveling to Ireland to continue his training at the large Dublin maternity hospital. However, in February 1847—after only four months—Breit was named professor of obstetrics at the university in Tübingen and the way was open for Semmelweis to function again as Klein's assistant.

Before resuming his duties, Semmelweis and two of his friends made an excursion to Venice. Semmelweis wrote, "I hoped the Venetian art treasures would revive my mind and spirits, which had been so seriously affected by my experiences in the maternity hospital."[9] He returned to Vienna on 20 March 1847 and immediately resumed his duties as assistant in the first section.

Upon returning, Semmelweis was shocked to learn that a friend, Professor Jakob Kolletschka, had died while he was away. Kolletschka's death proved to be a turning point in Semmelweis's work. Semmelweis gave the following description of Kolletschka's death and of its impact on his thinking:

> Kolletschka, professor of Forensic Medicine, often conducted autopsies for legal purposes in the company of students. During one such exercise, his finger was pricked by a student with the same knife that was being used in the autopsy. . . . Professor Kolletschka contracted lymphangitis and phlebitis in the upper extremity. Then, while I was still in Venice, he died of bilateral pleurisy, pericarditis, peritonitis, and meningitis. A few days before he died, a metastasis also formed in one eye. I was still animated by the art treasures of Venice, but the news of Kolletschka's death agitated me still more. In this excited condition I could see clearly that the disease from which Kolletschka died was identical to that from which so many hundred maternity patients had also died. The maternity patients also had lymphangitis, peritonitis, pericarditis, pleurisy, and meningitis; and metastases also formed in many of them. Day and night I was haunted by the image of Kolletschka's disease and was forced to recognize, ever more decisively, that the disease from which Kolletschka died was identical to that from which so many maternity patients died.
>
> . . . The cause of Professor Kolletschka's death was known; it was the wound by the autopsy knife that had been contaminated by cadaverous particles. Not the wound, but contamination of the wound by the cadaverous particles caused

his death. . . . I was forced to admit that if his disease was identical with the disease that killed so many maternity patients, then it must have originated from the same cause that brought it on in Kolletschka. In Kolletschka, the specific causal factor was the cadaverous particles that had been introduced into his vascular system. I was compelled to ask whether cadaverous particles had been introduced into the vascular systems of those patients whom I had seen die of this identical disease. I was forced to answer affirmatively.

Because of the anatomical orientation of the Viennese medical school, professors, assistants, and students have frequent opportunities to touch cadavers. Ordinary washing with soap is not sufficient to remove all adhering cadaverous particles. This is proven by the cadaverous smell that the hands retain for a longer or shorter time. In the examination of pregnant or delivering maternity patients, the hands, contaminated with cadaverous particles, are brought into contact with the genitals of these individuals, creating the possibility of resorption. With resorption, the cadaverous particles are introduced into the vascular system of the patient. In this way, maternity patients contract the same disease that was found in Kolletschka.[10]

Semmelweis realized that practices in the midwives' section were different. In contrast to the obstetrical students, student midwives ordinarily had no contact with cadavers. So here was a difference that could possibly explain the excessive mortality in the first section.

Semmelweis saw that this hypothesis might also explain other facts about childbed fever. For example, ordinarily there was no point in examining women who arrived at the hospital having already given birth, and as a result, women who delivered on the street were seldom examined. Thus, they were not exposed to the cadaverous poison that, as he thought, might be the cause of the disease, and they remained healthy. The relatively greater incidence of puerperal fever in winter months could be explained by the greater diligence of students in the winter: in summer "the charming surroundings of Vienna are more attractive than the reeking morgue or the sultry wards of the hospital."[11] Students who spent their time outside the morgue were less likely to convey cadaverous particles. Semmelweis could also explain why the mortality rate had been low during the years that Boer had directed the clinic and why it had become higher immediately after Klein was appointed: while Boer refused to allow his students to touch corpses, Klein required students to practice using cadavers of both women and fetuses.

It was clear why women delivering for the first time were particularly vulnerable to childbed fever. In a first delivery, the period of dilation was often extended. This meant that such women were examined more often by medical personnel and so were more likely to be exposed to cadaverous matter. Semmelweis could also see why the incidence of childbed fever had declined during the four months that Breit replaced him in the clinic and had then risen sharply after Breit left: Breit performed fewer autopsies than he did. Moreover, while the mortality rate did decline after the number of male students was reduced, this was because of there having been fewer autopsies being performed by the clinic personnel conducting examinations; it had nothing to do with the male students' supposed lack of gentleness. But Semmelweis also saw that his own diligence in performing autopsies had killed many of his patients: "Only God knows the number of patients who went prematurely to their graves because of me. I have examined corpses to an extent equaled by few other obstetricians."[12] Because Semmelweis could explain so many facts with his hypothesis, he was convinced he was on the right track.

Hours or even days after a physician or student would perform an autopsy, his hands bore a fetid smell from the death house. This smell was due to particles of decaying matter retained on the hands and around the nails and could not be removed by ordinary washing. Semmelweis concluded that some powerful cleaning agent was necessary—one that would destroy these particles. After considering other substances, he decided on a solution of chloride of lime as an effective and inexpensive disinfectant. Near the end of May 1847—about two months after returning from his vacation in Venice—Semmelweis (with Klein's permission) began requiring everyone in his section to wash thoroughly in the chlorine solution before examining patients. Immediately, the mortality rate in the first section dropped slightly below the rate in the second section.

Mortality remained low through June and July. However, in August a new group of students was admitted. Some of the students neglected the washings, and by the end of the month the mortality rate had increased once more. Semmelweis instituted stricter controls: one male student and one midwife were assigned to each woman in labor, and the names of these students were publicly displayed. In this way, Semmelweis could immediately identify anyone who neglected the washings.[13] Once again the mortality rate fell.

Semmelweis first concluded that cadaverous poisoning was the cause of the increased mortality in the first section. However, in the next few months he became persuaded that other sources of decaying organic matter were also dangerous: "In October 1847 a patient was admitted with a discharging medullary carcinoma of the uterus. She was assigned the bed at which the rounds were always initiated." One of Semmelweis's students later recalled that this woman was in confinement for several days and that, since her case "was highly interesting, everyone wished to examine her."[14]

> After examining this patient, those conducting the examination washed their hands with soap only. The consequence was that of twelve patients then delivering, eleven

died. The ichor from the discharging medullary carcinoma was not destroyed by soap and water. In the examinations, ichor was transferred to the remaining patients, and so childbed fever multiplied. Thus, childbed fever is caused not only by cadaverous particles adhering to the hands but also by ichor from living organisms. It is necessary to clean the hands with chlorine water, not only when one has been handling cadavers but also after examinations in which the hands could become contaminated with ichor. . . .

A new tragic experience persuaded me that air could also carry decaying organic matter. In November of the same year, an individual was admitted with a discharging carious left knee. In the genital region this person was completely healthy. Thus the examiners' hands presented no danger to the other patients. But the ichorous exhalations of the carious knee completely saturated the air of her ward. In this way the other patients were exposed and nearly all the patients in that room died.[15]

These two cases were important to Semmelweis's concept of childbed fever: from them, he inferred that exposure to any kind of decaying organic matter—not just cadaverous particles—could bring on the disease and that decaying organic matter could be conveyed in ways other than on the hands. By the late fall of 1847—about six months after he began the chlorine washings—Semmelweis was convinced that he understood the imbalance in mortality between the two sections and that conscientious washing with a chlorine solution could prevent the extra deaths.

Toward the end of 1847, accounts of Semmelweis's work began to spread around Europe. Semmelweis and his students wrote letters to the directors of several prominent maternity clinics; in these letters they described their recent observations. Ferdinand Hebra, Vienna's celebrated dermatologist and the editor of a leading Austrian medical journal, announced Semmelweis's discovery in the December 1847 and April 1848 issues of his periodical. Hebra claimed that Semmelweis's work had a practical significance comparable to that of Edward Jenner's introduction of cowpox inoculations to prevent smallpox.

A few obstetricians responded to these announcements, and the responses generally favored the use of chlorine washings. James Young Simpson, the most prominent British obstetrician, wrote back criticizing the Viennese for being so slow to adopt chlorine washings. He claimed that, in recognizing the danger of contagion, Semmelweis had only discovered what the British had recognized years earlier. Christian Bernard Tilanus from Amsterdam reported favorable results from washing in a chlorine solution. Gustav Adolph Michaelis, professor of obstetrics in Kiel, Germany, reported that his clinic had once been ravaged by child-bed fever but, since he had adopted chlorine washings, there had been no new cases of the disease. Somewhat later, Semmelweis learned that Michaelis had become convinced he was responsible for the death of his own cousin, whom he had delivered, because she had died of childbed fever. Michaelis became depressed and ended his own life by throwing himself under a train that was speeding into Hamburg.

In his letter, Michaelis also reported to Semmelweis that he had forwarded word of Semmelweis's discoveries to a colleague, Karl Edouard Marius Levy of Copenhagen. In a local medical periodical, Levy published an account of Semmelweis's work together with a critical response. Levy was not persuaded of the need for chlorine washings. He argued that "the amount of infective matter or vapor secluded around the fingernails could not be enough to kill a patient."[16]

One year after these first announcements—in the fall of 1848— a young British physician named C. H. F. Routh, who had been Semmelweis's student when the chlorine washings were initiated, wrote a lecture explaining Semmelweis's work. The lecture was presented before an important medical association in London and was published in a prominent medical journal. A few months later, another of Semmelweis's former students, M. F. Wieger, published a similar essay in a French periodical.

Thus, by the fall of 1848—within only eighteen months of his initial insight—Semmelweis had identified the cause of the excessive mortality in the first section of the obstetrical clinic, he had discovered how to reduce the mortality to the same favorable level that was maintained in the second section, and he had accumulated persuasive statistical evidence that his prophylaxis was safe and effective. Accounts of his discovery were being circulated throughout Europe. He had reason to expect that the chlorine washings would be widely adopted and that tens of thousands of lives would be saved. These were truly impressive accomplishments for a young and inexperienced physician—for someone who was nothing more than what, today, would be called a "head resident."

Unfortunately, there were already signs of trouble. The first such sign was that physicians who were responding to the early announcements of Semmelweis's work had misinterpreted his claims. Simpson, for instance, saw no difference between Semmelweis's view and the old British idea that childbed fever could be contagious. In fact, Semmelweis was warning against *all* decaying organic matter—not just against a specific contagion that originated from victims of childbed fever itself. This misunderstanding, and others like it, occurred partly because Semmelweis's work was known only through secondhand reports written by his colleagues and students. At this crucial stage, Semmelweis himself published nothing. The misinterpretations that followed these first announcements continued to cloud discussions of his work throughout the century.

The second alarming sign was political: just as Semmelweis's work was being announced by his students and colleagues, Europe was slipping into a period of exceptional political turbulence. Such conditions are not conducive to the disinterested evaluation of evidence and arguments.

In February 1848—two months after Ferdinand Hebra's first editorial announcing Semmelweis's discovery—riots broke out in Paris. The unrest quickly spread to other parts of Europe. On 13 March 1848 students from the University of Vienna demonstrated in favor of increased civil rights, including trial by jury, freedom of expression, and especially freedom of learning at the university. The Viennese demonstration was led by medical students and by young faculty members from the college of medicine. Workers from the suburbs soon joined the demonstration, and the situation grew progressively more ominous. Within hours, the Hapsburgs were forced to make concessions.

In the evening of the same day on which the demonstrations began, the Hapsburgs dismissed Clemens von Metternich, the detested prime minister; they decreed that students would be allowed to form a national guard intended to preserve the peace in Vienna and to protect the civil rights of the populace; and they granted relative independence and self-regulation to the faculties of higher education.

In Hungary, a strong movement for nationalistic reform and independence was already under way. Upon hearing that Metternich had fallen, the Hungarian Diet—led by the eloquent and courageous Lajos Kossuth—demanded the establishment of a national government and of a parliament to be elected by general male franchise. The Hapsburgs quickly granted these demands, but this did not stem the unrest. The Hungarian nationalists became progressively bolder, and many called for complete independence from the Hapsburg empire. However, Hungary contained large populations of Romanians, Croats, Serbs, and Slovaks; and these minorities feared that Hungarian independence would thwart their own nationalistic ambitions and threaten the rights they enjoyed within the empire. They opposed independence from Austria and issued demands of their own. Violence swept the country.

In Vienna, the March riots were followed by months of general unrest. Many of the affairs of ordinary life—including classroom instruction at the university—were impossible. The Hapsburgs remained in power, but they lived in constant fear of touching off further revolts in Vienna. By October, matters appeared to have stabilized, and the government felt secure enough to move against the Hungarian uprising; an army was ordered into Hungary to restore control. However, many Viennese were sympathetic to the Hungarian cause, and this new act of suppression touched off further violence in the city. Students demonstrated, and a few military units refused to march against the Hungarians. Yet, most of the army remained loyal to the Hapsburgs. The Viennese insurrection was quelled when the army bombarded the city with cannons. In the spring of 1849, Hapsburg armies—assisted by two-hundred thousand Russian troops—overwhelmed the Hungarians and reestablished Hapsburg control. The concessions that had been granted in the spring were withdrawn, and the leaders of the independence movement were imprisoned, exiled, or executed.

Historians disagree about Semmelweis's involvement in the Viennese uprisings and about whether the political events of 1848 influenced his subsequent career. All that is known about the first topic is easy to state: some of Semmelweis's brothers were punished for active participation in the Hungarian independence movement, and one must assume that Semmelweis himself was sympathetic to the cause. There is anecdotal evidence that he joined the National Guard of Vienna, and fifty years later a Swiss physician who had been Semmelweis's student reminisced that Semmelweis often appeared in his National Guard uniform.[17] Beyond this, there is no clear evidence that Semmelweis participated personally in the stormy events of 1848.

Although he seems not to have taken an active part in the Viennese riots, contemporary political developments were destined to have a profound, if indirect, influence on his career. Semmelweis's chief, Johannes Klein, was a conservative Austrian who, no doubt, was unsympathetic to the independence movements spreading through Hungary and in other parts of the empire. Like many other senior physicians and administrators, Klein saw the increased autonomy of the university as an erosion of traditional values and respect for authority, and he was skeptical of foreign democratic ideals.

Two years earlier, near the end of 1846, Klein had reduced the number of male physicians studying in the obstetrical clinic from forty-two to twenty and had limited the number of non-Austrian students in the clinic to a maximum of two.[18] Klein had justified this change on the grounds that foreigners were less careful in conducting examinations and were therefore more dangerous to the health of patients than were native Austrians. It is difficult not to see this action as a manifestation of Klein's dislike of everything foreign. Given the turbulence in Hungary, it seems likely that Klein mistrusted Semmelweis and that their conflicting political sentiments were a source of mutual animosity. But any hostility on this personal level was swallowed up in more immediate sources of conflict that divided the Viennese medical faculty just at the time Semmelweis's work was being announced.

In January 1849—twenty months after Semmelweis had begun the chlorine washings—Josef Skoda proposed that the medical faculty select a commission to investigate "the causes of the previously high and currently so meaningfully reduced mortality rate" in the first section of the obstetrical clinic.[19] Skoda's proposal was unanimously accepted by the faculty. Even Klein voted in favor of choosing the commission. Klein probably assumed that, as professor of obstetrics, he would himself be selected to serve as a member of the commission. However, when the commission was elected it consisted of Karl Rokitansky, Franz Schuh, and Josef Skoda.

In the next faculty meeting, Klein protested against Skoda's proposal. In explaining his objections, Klein observed that Skoda and the other elected members of the commission had shown themselves to be his personal enemies. Under these conditions,

Klein insisted, work carried out in his clinic could not be evaluated fairly and impartially.

Klein maintained that it was his prerogative as professor of obstetrics to appraise work conducted in his own clinic and that he fully intended to examine the effectiveness of the chlorine washings. A commission of outsiders—such as those who had been elected—would only be meddling in affairs about which they had no special knowledge or training, and such an investigation would certainly disrupt his clinic. Klein insisted that Skoda had shown himself to be his personal enemy and that Skoda's real motive for proposing the commission was that it would serve Skoda's own interests and those of his faction within the faculty.[20]

A central issue in the ensuing debate was whether the medical faculty actually had the authority to institute, on its own initiative, an investigation of the kind that Skoda had proposed. Skoda, Rokitansky, and other progressive young faculty members assumed that this authority was included among the concessions that the Hapsburgs had granted a few months earlier. But the conservative faction, led by Klein, vigorously disputed this assumption. Klein pointed out that all previous commissions had been initiated by the university administration—not by the faculty—and that nothing in the language of the concessions justified the faculty's action in assuming this new prerogative.

Because of this difference in interpretation, the election of the commission became a test case for measuring the real power and autonomy of the medical faculty. To resolve matters, Klein and his friends appealed to the administrative authorities. Not surprisingly, the authorities ruled that the faculty was not empowered to initiate the investigation; they overturned Skoda's proposal, and Klein was victorious.

In this affair, Klein's opposition did not focus on Semmelweis's ideas about childbed fever or even on Semmelweis's personal political sentiments, but rather on the reform movement within the university—a movement that Skoda and Rokitansky ardently supported and for which the proposed commission became a symbol. However, once Semmelweis and his work were drawn into this political dispute, it must have been quite obvious to everyone how Klein would react toward his Hungarian assistant. Even Skoda must have seen that, by using Semmelweis to attack Klein, he was exposing Semmelweis to personal and professional disaster.

Semmelweis's two-year appointment in the first section had begun in March 1846. In December 1848—one month before Skoda proposed forming the investigative commission—Semmelweis applied for a two-year extension so that he could continue his research. Such extensions were frequently awarded; indeed, Semmelweis's predecessor in the first section, his contemporary in the second section, and his successor in the first section all extended their original appointments in just this way. At first, Klein responded favorably to the idea of extending Semmelweis's appointment. However, Semmelweis did not continue to enjoy Klein's support.

On 20 January 1849, the very day on which Klein first protested against Skoda's proposal, a young physician named Carl Braun also applied for the position of assistant in the first section—possibly at Klein's own invitation. Semmelweis and Braun were the only two applicants for the post; and since Braun had received almost no special training in obstetrics, Semmelweis was obviously the better qualified. Semmelweis's application was supported by Skoda and Rokitansky and by most of the medical faculty. But—not surprisingly—Klein favored Braun. Since professors were ordinarily allowed to choose their own assistants, Braun received the appointment. On 20 March 1849 Semmelweis's term expired, and he was obliged to abandon his work in the obstetrical clinic.

Notes

1. György Gortvay and Imre Zoltán, *Semmelweis: His Life and Work* (Budapest, Hungary: Akadémiai Kiadó, 1968), p. 38.

2. A notice of the death of Carl Mayrhofer, signed "r," *Wiener medizinische Blätter* 5 (1882): col. 725.

3. Ignaz Semmelweis, *The Etiology, Concept, and Prophylaxis of Childbed Fever*, ed. and trans. K. Codell Carter (Madison: University of Wisconsin, 1983), p. 70. In this passage, and in several below, I have made slight adjustments in the terminology of my earlier translation.

4. Semmelweis, p. 86.

5. Semmelweis, p. 69.

6. Semmelweis, p. 73.

7. Semmelweis, p. 87.

8. Semmelweis, pp. 71–73.

9. Semmelweis, p. 87.

10. Semmelweis, pp. 87–89.

11. Semmelweis, p. 122.

12. Semmelweis, p. 98.

13. Friedrich Wieger, "Des moyens prophylactiques mis en usage au grand hôpital de Vienne contre l'apparition de la fièvre puerpérale," *Gazette médicale de Strasbourg* 9 (1849): cols. 97–105, at col. 100.

14. Franz Hektor Arneth, "Evidence of Puerperal Fever Depending on the Contagious Inoculation of Morbid Matter," *Monthly Journal of Medical Science* 12 (1851): 505–511, at p. 510.

15. Semmelweis, p. 93.

16. Quoted in Semmelweis, p. 183.

17. Gortvay and Zoltán, p. 63.

18. Semmelweis, p. 84.

19. Erna Lesky, *Ignaz Philipp Semmelweis und die Wiener medizinische Schule* (Vienna: Hermann Böhlaus, 1964), p. 21.

20. Lesky, pp. 23 f.

4

Resorption Fever

After attempting unsuccessfully to renew his assignment as Klein's assistant, Semmelweis petitioned the Viennese authorities to be appointed docent of obstetrics. A docent was a private lecturer who taught students and who had access to some university facilities, but who was paid by the students themselves rather than by the university. At first, because of Klein's opposition, Semmelweis's petition was denied. He reapplied, but the authorities delayed action on his request for more than a year.

While awaiting the results of his petition, Semmelweis conducted experiments—at Skoda's suggestion—in which the genitals of newly delivered rabbits were brushed with blood and other fluids from human corpses. Most of the rabbits died, and dissection revealed remains similar to those found in victims of childbed fever.

In October 1849, two months after Semmelweis concluded his animal experiments, Josef Skoda delivered a lecture on Semmelweis's work.[1] Skoda's purpose was supposedly to describe Semmelweis's discovery; unfortunately, he also took the opportunity to attack the obstetricians at the University of Prague. According to Skoda, women in the Prague maternity clinic were dying from childbed fever because the medical staff in Prague were examining their patients without first cleaning their hands. Skoda insisted that these deaths could be avoided if the obstetricians in Prague would only follow Semmelweis's example and require the use of chlorine washings.

Two obstetricians from the University of Prague, Wilhelm Friedrich Scanzoni and Bernhard Seyfert, responded to Skoda. They were outraged by his suggestion that childbed fever in their clinic was due to their own carelessness and denied that cadaverous poisoning was causing puerperal fever at their facility.[2] They also claimed to have tried chlorine washings, but reported that the procedure had not significantly reduced the incidence of the disease. Somewhat later, a medical student from Prague gave the following account of how chlorine washings were used in Seyfert's maternity clinic:

> Seyfert wanted to provide the clinical students with conclusive proof that the washings were entirely useless and that it was impossible to imagine that the infection of maternity patients with cadaverous matter resulted in the [diseased] puerperal state. One must realize that most of the examining students came directly from the morgue and so it was easy for cadaverous matter to be conveyed in this way. In fact, in spite of the so-called washings, the disease did not become less frequent or less intense in the institution. But for me this was no proof against the views of Dr. Semmelweis, because I saw with my own eyes that there was usually nothing resembling a true washing of the hands. Usually, only the fingertips were dipped once into an opaque fluid that had served the same purpose for many days and that was itself completely saturated with harmful matter. Many of the gentlemen finally abandoned even this manipulation and used only ordinary water, often even without soap.[3]

Almost three years had now elapsed since Semmelweis had initiated the chlorine washings. In those years, Semmelweis—

who said of himself that he sought to avoid all controversy—
had become the focus of a fierce power struggle within the
Vienna medical faculty, and his work had become the subject
of a bitter dispute among European obstetricians. Josef Skoda
had provoked both controversies by using Semmelweis's work as
a basis for attacking his own enemies. Remarkably, Semmelweis
himself had yet to give a lecture or publish a paper on his own
work.

On 15 May 1850, seven months after Skoda's lecture, Semmelweis finally presented his findings before the Imperial Viennese
Society of Physicians. The discussion of his lecture continued
through three successive meetings in June and July. Although
the lecture was not published, apparently because Semmelweis
did not take the time to write it out, the secretary's minutes of
the lecture and of the subsequent discussions were published.[4]
In his lecture, Semmelweis claimed that every case of childbed
fever—without a single exception—occurred when decaying organic
matter was resorbed (literally, absorbed back) into the living
tissues of maternity patients. Because he believed that this was
the only way in which the disease ever came about, Semmelweis
referred to childbed fever as a "resorption fever."

As we have seen, other accounts of puerperal fever (like standard accounts of most diseases at the time) attributed the disease
to many different and unrelated causes. By contrast, Semmelweis
insisted that overeating, immorality, fear, chilling, and all the
other causes that obstetricians identified were all beside the point;
all that mattered was absolute cleanliness. From our vantage
point, Semmelweis's claim seems utterly reasonable. However, at
the time, it was directly opposed to what everyone else thought
about disease causation in general. By adopting this extreme view,
Semmelweis made a radical break with existing medical thought—
one that separated him from almost every other physician in
Europe.

In the July meeting, Eduard Lumpe argued against several of Semmelweis's claims. Lumpe had preceded Franz Breit as Johann Klein's assistant in the first section; and Lumpe's own thorough study of childbed fever had been published five years earlier in 1845, the year before Semmelweis became Klein's assistant. In that paper, Lumpe mentioned virtually all the evidence Semmelweis was now using to support his new concept of the disease, yet Lumpe did not believe this evidence implied that every case of childbed fever had the same one cause. While Lumpe was willing to grant the usefulness of chlorine washings, he emphatically rejected Semmelweis's concept of the disease. Lumpe wrote:

> I was originally overjoyed as I heard of the fortunate results of the chlorine washings—as anyone must have been who has had the misfortune of witnessing so many blossoming young individuals fall, as so many unnerved fragile wrecks, before this devastating plague. However, during my two years as assistant in the first section, I observed such enormous variations in the incidence of illness and death that I must doubt the [supposed] origin and prophylaxis currently in vogue.[5]

After many detailed criticisms of Semmelweis, Lumpe concluded:

> If adopting the washings makes it possible to avoid even the least significant of the many concurring factors that cause puerperal fever, then their initial adoption was a sufficiently great service. Whether this is in fact the case, only the future can decide. In the meantime, I believe we should wait and wash.[6]

Following Lumpe's lecture, a few physicians commented favorably on the chlorine washings although there is no evidence in the published minutes that anyone in Vienna supported Semmelweis's claim that childbed fever was invariably caused by contamination. Apparently neither Josef Skoda nor Ferdinand Hebra made any comments whatsoever in the discussion of Semmelweis's lecture.

Over the next several months, no new developments and no further public discussions related to Semmelweis's work. Lumpe's critical essay was the only published response to Semmelweis's lecture.

Five months later, in October 1850, Semmelweis was finally appointed docent of obstetrics. However, the terms of the appointment refused him access to cadavers and limited him to teaching students by using leather fabricated models only.

A few days after being notified of his appointment, Semmelweis left Vienna abruptly and returned to Budapest—apparently without so much as saying good-bye to his former friends and colleagues. Semmelweis himself explained that he left Vienna because he was unable to endure further frustrations in dealing with the Viennese medical establishment. During his last year in Vienna, he had been drawn into two major controversies when the developments in the first section of the maternity clinic were used by Skoda to attack Skoda's own enemies. The response to Semmelweis's lecture had been skeptical and unsympathetic; and so far as one can tell from the published record, he received no support from Skoda or from any other supposed friends. After Semmelweis's lecture, there seems to have been no further discussion of his views about childbed fever, and the terms of his appointment as docent denied him access to the facilities necessary for further research. Given all of this, Semmelweis's sudden departure from Vienna seems entirely reasonable, if not totally justified.

In the fall of 1850, Budapest was somber and depressed. Eighteen months earlier, Hapsburg armies had violently suppressed the Hungarian revolution. In the process, they had destroyed parts of the city. When Semmelweis returned from Vienna, life had still not returned to normal.

Several prominent Budapest physicians had actively participated in the Hungarian independence movement. When order was restored, they were punished by the Hapsburg authorities. János Balassa, the most famous surgeon in Hungary, was temporarily removed from his professorship and imprisoned while other prominent physicians were required to suspend their practices for several months. Hungarian intellectuals hated everything associated with the Hapsburgs. By contrast, Semmelweis seems to have taken no active part in the rebellion. He returned to Budapest having just been appointed docent of obstetrics, an appointment that indicated the Viennese authorities judged him politically safe. Under these circumstances it is not surprising that Semmelweis encountered a cool reception in Budapest. He did not find immediate employment, and he was not quickly accepted as a colleague or friend.

In the spring of 1851, several months after returning to Budapest, Semmelweis was finally given a relatively insignificant position as the unpaid director of a small maternity facility in St. Rochus Hospital. This quaint baroque hospital is still in operation near the center of Pest. It has since been renamed in Semmelweis's honor, and a large statue of Semmelweis has been erected directly in front of its main entrance.

Before Semmelweis's appointment, the maternity clinic at the St. Rochus Hospital, under the direction of a surgeon, had been seriously afflicted with childbed fever. Since no students were trained in the hospital and since few autopsies were performed there, no one saw that Semmelweis's discoveries in Vienna were relevant to the problem. However, upon visiting the hospital, Semmelweis immediately saw what was wrong: the surgeon who directed the maternity facility examined patients while his hands were still caked with blood and tissues from his surgical procedures. Once Semmelweis was appointed director, the surgeon no longer examined the patients. Semmelweis ordered the facility cleaned and immediately adopted chlorine washings. The mortality rate fell just as it had in Vienna's General Hospital.

In spite of his success, Semmelweis's ideas were not accepted by the other obstetricians in Budapest. While Semmelweis was working at St. Rochus Hospital, Ede Flórián Birly was professor of obstetrics at the University of Pest. He never adopted Semmelweis's methods. Birly died three years later in 1854, and it then became necessary for the medical faculty to nominate several candidates from whom the Viennese authorities could select Birly's successor. Semmelweis applied for the position, but he received fewer votes from his Hungarian colleagues than did Carl Braun— Semmelweis's successor as Klein's assistant and his bitter enemy.[7] In the end, Semmelweis was appointed as Birly's successor, but only because the Viennese authorities overruled the wishes of the Hungarians. The authorities did this on the grounds that only someone who spoke Hungarian could possibly direct the obstetrical clinic in Pest, and Braun did not speak Hungarian. In this way the Hapsburgs forced Semmelweis on his unwilling compatriots.

As professor of obstetrics, Semmelweis instituted chlorine washings at the University of Pest maternity clinic. He insisted that bed linen and all obstetrical equipment and supplies be disinfected before use. Once again he attained impressive results.

Semmelweis had now achieved dramatic successes at three obstetrical facilities. By following strict disinfection procedures, he achieved success in gynecological surgeries that were prohibitively dangerous at other hospitals around Europe. Even so, his ideas continued to be ridiculed and rejected both in Vienna and in Budapest. In 1856, Semmelweis's assistant, József Fleischer reported the success of the new chlorine washings in a prominent Viennese medical periodical. At the conclusion of the report, the Viennese editor added these sentences: "We believe that this chlorine-washing theory has long outlived its usefulness. The experiences and statistical results of most maternity institutions protest against the views presented above. It is time we are no longer to be deceived by this theory."[8]

In 1857 Semmelweis married Mária Weidenhoffer, the beautiful daughter of a successful merchant in Pest. At the time of their marriage, Mária was eighteen and Ignaz was thirty-nine. The couple moved into an apartment in a building on Váci utca, a short walk from the facilities where Semmelweis worked.

In the nineteenth century, Váci utca was an important shopping street. Today it is a noisy and active pedestrian zone, lined with shops that cater especially to tourists. The ground floor of the building in which the Semmelweis family lived is now a bookstore, and a small commemorative plaque to Semmelweis hangs in a front window. The building encloses a quiet courtyard from which an ancient well-worn circular marble stairway ascends to the third floor, where the Semmelweis apartment was located.

Semmelweis and his wife had five children: a son who died shortly after birth; a daughter who died at four months; a second daughter who lived to adulthood, but who remained unmarried; a second son who took his own life at the age of twenty-three, probably as a consequence of gambling debts; and finally, a third daughter—the only one of the Semmelweis children who married and had children of her own.

Semmelweis had delivered his lecture on childbed fever in May 1850 and had left Vienna in the following October. By the time of his marriage in 1857, he had still not published an account of his own research. Nevertheless, his opinions continued to be discussed in European medical literature. While some of those who responded to Semmelweis acknowledged chlorine washings could be useful, by 1859 no one accepted his concept of the disease. Whatever the other physicians may have believed about the need for chlorine disinfection, Semmelweis stood entirely alone in respect to his claim that every case of childbed fever had one common cause.

In 1858 Semmelweis finally published his own account of his work in a short essay, "The Etiology of Childbed Fever." This led to a flurry of publications. Two years later he published a second essay, "The Difference in Opinion between Myself and the English Physicians regarding Childbed Fever." In October 1860 he published his only book, *The Etiology, Concept, and Prophylaxis of Childbed Fever.* In 1861, when his book did not have the impact that he had hoped, Semmelweis began publishing a series of open letters bitterly attacking various prominent obstetricians. He also explained his views in a letter written in English that appeared in a British periodical.

The account of childbed fever that is set forth in these publications rests on a new definition. Semmelweis defined "childbed fever" as "a resorption fever determined through the resorption of decaying animal-organic matter."[9] From this definition, it follows that every case of childbed fever has the same one cause, namely, the resorption of decaying animal-organic matter. Semmelweis calculated that, in approximately 1 percent of all deliveries, decaying organic matter was generated within the birth canal of the delivering women: this occurred when tissues were damaged or when fluids or fragments of the placenta were retained in the uterus. While Semmelweis believed that childbed fever was unavoidable in such cases, he was convinced that all other cases of the disease arose when decaying organic matter was introduced into the vascular systems of patients, usually on the hands of medical personnel. This meant that by washing in a disinfectant solution (thereby destroying the decaying organic matter) one could reduce the incidence of the disease to about 1 percent. This was approximately the level of morbidity that Semmelweis achieved in his own practice.

To Semmelweis's contemporaries, his new definition of the disease looked like a semantic trick. By limiting attention to cases that shared the one common cause, Semmelweis appeared simply to be defining most cases of childbed fever out of existence. His concept of childbed fever seemed to trivialize the quest for control of the disease.

Christopher Columbus—while arguing with skeptics, who did not believe that one could reach China by sailing west from Europe—is said to have challenged his opponents to make an egg stand upright on a table. When they were unable to do so, Columbus seized the egg and smashed it onto the table, where it remained standing. The egg of Columbus has become a metaphor for any attempt to solve an intractable problem by disregarding the implicit conditions upon which it depends. This is exactly what Semmelweis appeared to be doing with his new definition of "childbed fever." Eduard Lumpe observed: "When one thinks how, since the first occurrence of puerperal fever epidemics, observers of all times have sought in vain for its causes and the means of preventing it, Semmelweis's theory takes on the appearance of the egg of Columbus."[10]

Yet, remarkably, Semmelweis's approach was exactly the kind of redefinition required to rationalize practical medicine. If diseases could be caused in different and essentially unrelated ways, then no single prophylaxis or therapy could be consistently effective. For example, in the early nineteenth century, "hydrophobia" (rabies) had been defined as an intense inability to swallow. This condition could be caused in several ways—for example, by psychological disorders, by blows to the throat, or by the bites of rabid dogs. Under these circumstances, treatment that might have been effective in some cases would be totally useless in other cases of the same disease. This made therapy so confusing that no systematic measures could ever be discovered. To find such measures, investigators needed to redefine diseases so that each had only one constant cause.

Clearly this was a problem in the treatment of childbed fever. Nineteenth-century physicians believed the very treatment required in some cases of the disease could itself provoke the disorder. Fever was often ascribed to excessive consumption, and the favored treatment was removing blood. But an inadequate diet was also believed to be a possible cause of the disease, and charity patients were malnourished. Thus, before they could be bled, charity patients were strengthened by being fed nourishing foods. This meant that the first step in treating a charity patient—feeding her—could exacerbate the very inflammation the physician was trying to combat. Physicians warned that treatment must be carefully adapted to the condition of each individual patient. As one practitioner observed, "Only the best physicians of all times have realized that similar cases of the most different diseases require the same treatment and that different cases of the same disease require different treatments. Conditions, rather than the disease, must be the basis for determination."[11] But it was impossible to say exactly which conditions were relevant to making the determination. As a result, treatment was inconsistent and confusing; effective practical medicine was all but impossible. Defining diseases so that each had only one specific cause was an essential step in the development of effective techniques for controlling any disease. Ignaz Semmelweis was among the first to adopt this approach.[12]

Semmelweis's book was published in 1860 when he was forty-two years old. He expected his book to save the lives of thousands of women who delivered in the maternity clinics of Europe, but the book was ignored and had little impact on contemporary obstetrical practice. Semmelweis was outraged at the callous indifference of the medical profession and began publishing open letters in which he denounced several prominent European obstetricians as irresponsible murderers. Even before this time, Semmelweis had not been held in high regard by his peers. These letters further undermined his professional credibility.

Semmelweis had always expressed himself freely and enthusiastically. Now he turned every conversation to the topic of childbed fever, and he spoke without taking into account those people who may have overheard him. During the summer of 1865, his public behavior became irritating and embarrassing to his associates and family. He also began to drink immoderately; he spent progressively more time away from his family, sometimes in the company of a prostitute; and his wife noticed changes in his sexual behavior. On 13 July 1865 the Semmelweis family visited friends, and during the visit Semmelweis's behavior seemed particularly inappropriate. As they returned home, it suddenly occurred to Mária that her husband was losing his mind. The next day she confided in Lajos Markusovsky, a Budapest physician who had been Semmelweis's friend since the days when they were medical students together in Vienna.

During the next week, Semmelweis attended a regular meeting of the Pest College of Medical Professors. According to one account, when Semmelweis was called on to make a routine report, "he rose, took a piece of paper from his trousers pocket and, to the stupefaction of those present, began to read the text of the midwives' oath."[13] This anecdote is invariably cited as conclusive proof that Semmelweis had become insane. However, the author of the account was not himself present at the meeting, and there is no corroboration for the story, which first appeared in print seven years after the alleged event. Moreover, while Semmelweis's name appears twice in the official minutes of the meeting, no comments in the minutes indicate his behavior was in any way unusual. During the meeting, Semmelweis applied for an increase in salary. Within a few days, the increase was approved both by the medical faculty and by the university administrators—developments difficult to understand if his behavior had, in fact, been as inappropriate as the anecdote suggests. The story may be based on some actual occurrence, but it probably gives a false impression of what actually took place.

Semmelweis does seem to have recognized that his health was failing. A few days after the faculty meeting, at his own request, he was examined by a friend and fellow physician, János Bókai. Bókai, a pediatrician and the director of a children's hospital in Budapest, recorded that, until recently, nothing had been observed "that could be judged as an anomalous expression of [Semmelweis's] mental life. His reasoning was always correct and consistent, his judgment according to his motivations correct; he defended his scientific views with a passion bordering on fanaticism, but with continual consistency in his opinion and in his motivation."[14] For about five weeks, however, the Semmelweis family had been noticing "that his expression and actions were different from his earlier habits." Bókai then mentioned some of the changes in behavior that Mária Semmelweis had earlier observed.

Today, it is impossible to appraise the nature or the seriousness of Semmelweis's disorder. All the recorded symptoms are compatible with several different interpretations. Semmelweis could have been showing early signs of progressive paralysis—tertiary syphilis. Or he could have been emotionally exhausted from overwork and stress. In the nineteenth century, exhaustion was treated by a few weeks' rest in a sanitarium. And indeed, following the examination, Semmelweis made plans to travel to a spa at Gräfenberg in southern Germany for the purpose of undergoing water treatments.

At this point, events took a dramatic and perhaps sinister turn. On 29 July 1865, János Balassa, professor of practical surgery at the University of Pest, wrote a referral committing Semmelweis to a Viennese insane asylum. Contemporary regulations required that such referrals be signed by three physicians. The referral to commit Semmelweis was signed first by a local internist named János Wagner, then by Balassa, and finally by János Bókai, the pediatrician who had examined Semmelweis. Balassa seems to have been hostile to Semmelweis ever since Semmelweis returned to Budapest in 1850; in any event, neither Balassa nor Wagner was among his friends. No evidence exists that either physician examined or interviewed Semmelweis before signing the order. None of the three physicians was trained in psychiatry. Although there were respected psychiatrists in Budapest, not one of them was consulted.

Given the imperfect historical record, it is impossible to decide whether the decision to have Semmelweis committed was justified. This much seems clear: Semmelweis's shrill and progressively more outrageous attacks on the European medical establishment had become embarrassing to everyone around him. Neither his medical colleagues nor his merchant in-laws would have been reluctant to have him silenced. Once Semmelweis began showing signs of instability, these signs may have been quickly—even prematurely— exploited as grounds for having him committed.

On the evening of the same day the commitment order was signed, 29 July 1865, Semmelweis left Budapest—supposedly on the first leg of his trip to the spa at Gräfenberg. He was accompanied by his wife, an unweaned infant daughter, his wife's uncle, and one of his assistants. The first stage of the journey took the party to Vienna by an overnight train. On the following morning, a Sunday, they were met at the Vienna train station by Semmelweis's former colleague and friend Ferdinand Hebra, the prominent dermatologist.

At the station, following a plan that had been arranged in advance, Hebra persuaded Semmelweis to interrupt his trip temporarily and make a short visit to what was purported to be Hebra's own sanitarium in Vienna. While the rest of the party waited with Hebra's wife, Hebra and the uncle took Semmelweis directly to an insane asylum located in Lazarettgasse, not far from the General Hospital. The asylum there was a large public institution—definitely not among Vienna's best.

Upon arrival at the asylum, Semmelweis was neither examined nor interviewed, and no attempt was made to determine whether he actually required confinement. Hebra and the uncle soon managed to slip away. Semmelweis surmised what was happening and tried to escape. A fight ensued in which Semmelweis was severely beaten by several guards. He was secured in a straitjacket and confined within a darkened cell. The next morning his wife came to the asylum to visit him but was told by the director that a visit would be impossible.

Semmelweis remained in the asylum for about two weeks. A medical record was kept, but this strange document raises more questions than it answers. There is no indication who observed him, who was in charge of his care, or even who compiled the medical record itself. Nowhere in the entire document is there a single reference that would identify anyone professionally associated with Semmelweis while he was in the asylum. There is no indication that Semmelweis was examined or treated by specialists, although there are three incidental allusions to unnamed physicians. Aside from the straitjacket, the only references to treatment involve superficial measures like dousing him with cold water and administering castor oil. Any medical facts given about Semmelweis, such as his pulse rate and temperature, are always given in round numbers and are often only estimated.

Because this medical record was written so carelessly, is so superficial, and contains inconsistencies and modifications, one modern biographer has conjectured that the entire account of Semmelweis's fifteen days in the asylum may have been hastily sketched out from memory *after* Semmelweis died.[15]

Early on, the medical record does mention a serious wound in the middle finger of Semmelweis's right hand. Since Bókai did not mention this wound in the account of his examination of Semmelweis, it may have been inflicted on Semmelweis by the asylum guards. Over the days Semmelweis remained in the institution, the anonymous recorder noted that the wound became gangrenous—there is no indication Semmelweis received any treatment for the condition. As the days passed, Semmelweis, unable to sleep, gradually became weaker and delirious. Boils spread over his extremities. Ignaz Semmelweis died in the evening of 13 August 1865 at the age of forty-seven. Although it had been obvious for hours that he was dying and though the medical record clearly indicated that he was Roman Catholic, no priest was called to administer the last rites.

Semmelweis's body was taken to the pathological institute of the Vienna General Hospital—to the same dissection rooms where he himself had conducted autopsies each morning in his quest for the cause of childbed fever. The autopsy of Semmelweis, supervised and possibly performed by Karl Rokitansky, revealed extensive internal injuries that could have been sustained only in beatings to which he had been subjected in the asylum. The cause of death was identified as pyemia—blood poisoning. Semmelweis had been severely beaten by the asylum guards and then left essentially untreated until his numerous wounds became infected and he died of blood poisoning—one of the diseases that, in maternity patients, would have been called childbed fever.

Semmelweis was buried in Vienna on 15 August 1865. Only a few persons attended the services, and most of those in attendance were from the Vienna General Hospital. These included Karl Rokitansky and two of Semmelweis's bitter enemies, the brothers Carl and Gustav Braun. From Budapest, only Semmelweis's friend Lajos Markusovsky attended the funeral. Not one family member, not one in-law, not one colleague from the University of Pest was in attendance. Semmelweis's wife later explained her own absence on the grounds that, after her husband was committed, she became so ill she had been unable to leave her bed for six weeks.[16]

A few Viennese medical periodicals included brief announcements of Semmelweis's death. Two periodicals promised to provide longer eulogies in later issues, but neither promise was kept.

The Budapest periodical *Orvosi Hetilap*, edited at the time by Lajos Markusovsky, contained a brief notice of Semmelweis's death. Remarkably, since Markusovsky had himself attended the funeral, the notice indicates Semmelweis had been taken to Vienna on

20 July and had been buried there on 16 August—both dates were wrong.

Within two weeks of Semmelweis's death, the Hungarian Association of Physicians and Natural Scientists conducted an annual excursion; the group was led by János Balassa. The association rules specified that a commemorative address be delivered in honor of each member who had died in the preceding year. For Semmelweis there was no address; so far as one can judge from the records of the association, his death was never even mentioned. The statutes of the Pest Association of Physicians also required that a eulogy be delivered in honor of each member in the year of his death; in Semmelweis's case, seven years elapsed before this was done.[17]

Semmelweis had two assistants, and after his death they both applied for his teaching position. However, at the recommendation of János Balassa, a physician named János Diescher was appointed instead. Earlier in his career, Diescher had completed a course that qualified him to conduct deliveries, but he had never been trained in obstetrics. The extent to which he followed Semmelweis's use of chlorine washings is clear from what happened to the mortality rate at the Pest maternity clinic: as soon as Diescher took charge, mortality jumped to six percent—six times the rate Semmelweis had consistently maintained. But there were no inquiries and no protests; the physicians of Budapest said nothing. Almost no one—either in Vienna or in Budapest—seems to have been willing to acknowledge Semmelweis's life and work. "One said nothing of Semmelweis, it was almost as though one was ashamed of his memory."[18]

In 1891 Semmelweis's remains were moved to Budapest. On 11 October 1964 they were transferred once more, this time to a space in the internal courtyard wall of the house in Tabán in which he had been born.

Notes

1. Josef Skoda, "Über die von Dr. Semmelweis, entdeckte wahre Ursache der in der Wiener Gebäranstalt ungewöhnlich häufig vorkommenden Erkrankungen der Wöchnerinnen, und des Mittels zur Verminderung dieser Erkrankungen bis auf die gewöhnliche Zahl," *Zeitschrift der k. k. Gesellschaft der Ärzte zu Wien* 6, no. 1 (1850): 107–117.

2. Wilhelm Friedrich Scanzoni, "Über die von Dr. Semmelweis, entdeckte wahre Ursache der in der Wiener Gebäranstalt ungewöhnlich häufig vorkommenden Erkrankungen der Wöchnerinnen, und des Mittels zur Verminderung dieser Erkrankungen bis auf die gewöhnliche Zahl," and Bernhard Seyfert, "Ergänzende Bermerkungen zu dem vorstehenden Aufsatze," *Vierteljahrschrift für die praktische Heilkunde*, Literarischer Anzeiger 2 (1850): 25–33 and 34–36.

3. Georg Martius, "Mittheilungen aus den Kliniken zu Prag," *Ärztliches Intelligenzblatt* 4 (1857): 410–415, at pp. 410 f.

4. The minutes are reprinted in Tiberius von Györy, *Semmelweis' gesammelte Werke* (Jena, Germany: Gustav Fischer, 1905), pp. 49–58.

5. Eduard Lumpe, "Zur Theorie der Puerperalfieber," *Zeitschrift der k. k. Gesellschaft der Ärzte zu Wien* 2 (1850): 392–398, at p. 392.

6. Lumpe, p. 398.

7. György Gortvay and Imre Zoltán, *Semmelweis: His Life and Work* (Budapest, Hungary: Akadémiai Kiadó, 1968), p. 93.

8. József Fleischer, "Statistischer Bericht der Gebärklinik an der k. k. Universität zu Pest," *Wiener medizinische Wochenschrift* 6 (1856): cols. 534–536, at col. 536.

9. Ignaz Semmelweis, "Die Aetiologie des Kindbettfiebers," reprinted in von Györy, p. 70; Ignaz Semmelweis, *The Etiology, Concept, and Prophylaxis of Childbed Fever*, ed. and trans. K. Codell Carter (Madison: University of Wisconsin, 1983), p. 114.

10. Lumpe, p. 392.

11. Rudolf Virchow, *Gesammelte Abhandlungen zur wissenschaftlichen Medicin* (Frankfurt a. M., Germany: Meidinger, 1856), p. 34.

12. K. Codell Carter, "Semmelweis and His Predecessors," *Medical History* 25 (1981): 57–72.

13. Gortvay and Zoltán, p. 187.

14. K. Codell Carter, Scott Abbott, and James L. Siebach, "Five Documents Relating to the Final Illness and Death of Ignaz Semmelweis," *Bulletin of the History of Medicine*, forthcoming.

15. Georg Silló-Seidl, *Die Wahrheit über Semmelweis* (Geneva, Switzerland: Ariston, 1978), p. 198.

16. Silló-Seidl, p. 116.

17. István Benedek, *Semmelweis' Krankheit* (Budapest, Hungary: Akadémiai Kiadó, 1983), p. 87.

18. István Benedek, *Ignaz Philipp Semmelweis* (Vienna: Hermann Böhlaus, 1983), p. 320.

5

Mayrhofer's Discovery

About one hundred miles west of Vienna, a short distance south of Austria's main east-west Autobahn, is an ancient Benedictine monastery named Kremsmünster, founded in the eighth century. Its present buildings date from the seventeenth and eighteenth centuries, and, like most Austrian architectural monuments, they are predominantly baroque. The abbey is located in the hilly transition zone between the Danube basin to the northeast and the Austrian Alps to the southwest and is beautifully situated on the shoulder of a steep hill overlooking the Krems river. The hills surrounding the abbey are mostly covered with farms and pastures, but also with vineyards and isolated patches of pine forest.

In 1839 Karl Wilhelm Mayrhofer was appointed physician to the Kremsmünster abbey. Mayrhofer and his wife, Josepha Wildschgo Mayrhofer, moved into a large gray building located just outside the northern walls of the monastery. At the time, the couple had a son named Carl, who had been born two years earlier on 2 June 1837. As he grew older, Carl attended school in the abbey, where his teachers recognized that he was unusually bright. Following his father's example, Carl Mayrhofer went on to study medicine at the University of Vienna.

In 1860, the same year in which Semmelweis's book appeared, Mayrhofer was awarded an M.D. degree. After studying surgery for two additional years, he decided to specialize in obstetrics. In 1862 he was appointed second assistant to Carl Braun, who had replaced Johannes Klein as professor of obstetrics at the university. Thus, Mayrhofer began working in the first section of the Viennese maternity clinic—in the same facility where, fifteen years earlier, Semmelweis had instituted chlorine washings.

During the 1850s, in various books and articles, Carl Braun had identified thirty possible causes of childbed fever. Among these, he had given particular attention to the possibility of infection by airborne germs. In the 1850s, tissue decomposition, as is regularly observed in childbed fever, was believed to resemble organic fermentation; and the young French chemist Louis Pasteur had argued that fermentation occurred when a fermentable substance, such as grape juice, was invaded by airborne germs. This made it seem likely that childbed fever could also be caused by the invasion of germs. Semmelweis ridiculed Braun for trying to explain the disease in this way;[1] he insisted that airborne germs were irrelevant and that the disease always arose from the resorption of decaying animal-organic matter. At the time that Mayrhofer became Braun's assistant, Braun was intensely interested in this dispute. Mayrhofer later wrote: "[Professor Braun] encouraged me to the highest degree. He said he had such an interest in resolving the affair he would gladly cover the research costs from his own resources and make available to me, for this purpose, all the clinical materials [i.e., maternity patients and corpses]."[2] Braun probably expected that Mayrhofer would confirm his own views about the etiology of childbed fever.

Mayrhofer immediately began studying the possible role of microorganisms in the disease. Because childbed fever often seemed to originate in the uterus, Mayrhofer began looking for living organisms in the uterine discharges of puerperal fever victims. At first he found nothing, because the only microscope available in the Viennese obstetrical clinic was not powerful enough to make such organisms clearly visible. However, through Braun's efforts, a new instrument was procured, and Mayrhofer's search began to yield results. One year later, in 1863, he published his first paper.[3] Later in the same year, Mayrhofer delivered a lecture on childbed fever before the most prestigious medical association in Vienna. This lecture was also published.[4] Both of Mayrhofer's papers were abstracted and reviewed in Viennese medical periodicals.

In these two publications, Mayrhofer referred to earlier research on the role of microorganisms in certain animal diseases and to earlier conjectures that some infectious human diseases could be caused by microorganisms. He also cited Pasteur's research on fermentation. Mayrhofer reported having studied the uterine discharges of more than one hundred living and dead victims of childbed fever, and he characterized and classified the various organisms he found. He noted that they differed in size and shape, in their motility, in their reactions to acidic media, and in their capacities to ferment various liquids. Following common usage, Mayrhofer referred to all of these organisms as "vibrions."

Mayrhofer became particularly interested in a certain class of motile vibrions that were consistent in size, that were incapable of living in acids, and that fermented various sugar solutions. Mayrhofer reported that these vibrions were especially abundant in the uterine discharges of diseased patients. Sometimes he found the same organisms in healthy patients, but never until five days or more after delivery. He hypothesized that the normally acidic vaginal secretions of healthy patients protected them from invasion by these parasites.

Mayrhofer tried to decide whether vibrions actually caused childbed fever or whether the diseased patient simply provided a suitable medium in which they could flourish. To accumulate evidence of causation, Mayrhofer sprayed fluids containing organisms into the genitals of newly delivered rabbits. Most of the rabbits became diseased and died, and postmortem examinations revealed large numbers of the same vibrions as well as morbid changes similar to those in puerperal fever victims.

For more conclusive evidence of causality, Mayrhofer cultivated vibrions in a sugar and ammonia solution. After filtering the solution to isolate the vibrions from other decomposition products, he sprayed the vibrions into the rabbits' genitals. Again the rabbits died, and again Mayrhofer found the familiar morbid remains in their carcasses.

Mayrhofer's early work was based directly on Braun's concept of childbed fever, and his initial results were entirely compatible with Braun's views. Perhaps this contributed to the favorable reception that Mayrhofer's first publications received in Vienna.

By 1864 Braun had good reason to feel vindicated. His views seemed to be supported by Mayrhofer's discoveries. Another of Braun's students, August Theodor Stamm, presented papers in which he argued that improved ventilation, rather than the use of chlorine washings, was responsible for the favorable mortality rates in the first section of the clinic.[5] Braun himself published papers maintaining that proper ventilation was the most important prophylaxis against childbed fever.[6] On the strength of the accumulating evidence, Braun persuaded the Viennese authorities to install an expensive new ventilation system in the maternity clinic.

However, just as Braun seemed to be winning the dispute about the nature of childbed fever, further research led Mayrhofer to conclude Braun's concept of the disease was fundamentally wrong.

Toward the end of 1864 Mayrhofer delivered a second lecture on childbed fever. This lecture was published in 1865—the same year in which Semmelweis died in the Viennese insane asylum. It was to be Mayrhofer's last work on childbed fever.[7] After this lecture, Mayrhofer completely abandoned his innovative research on vibrions. Over the next several years, he published a few articles on various topics in obstetrics, but in only one passage did he ever again discuss childbed fever, and in that passage he merely reaffirmed his earlier claims about the disease.[8]

Mayrhofer's second lecture marked a turning point in his relations with Braun, and the reason is obvious. In this lecture, Mayrhofer rejected Braun's concept of childbed fever and adopted a position that was much closer to Semmelweis's view. Mayrhofer revealed his change of allegiance in two ways. First, although he had originally agreed with Braun that vibrion germs were usually conveyed through the air, in his second lecture, he gave up trying to explain how this could happen. While Mayrhofer left open the possibility of airborne germs, he concluded, exactly as Semmelweis had before him, that infection was usually due to the contaminated hands of examining physicians. This meant that chlorine washings were indispensable—a conclusion that was in direct opposition to Braun, who continued to insist that inadequate ventilation was a far more common cause of the disease.

Second, in his final lecture, Mayrhofer, like Semmelweis, identified a universal necessary cause for all cases of childbed fever. As in Semmelweis's account, the existence of such a cause followed from a new characterization of the disease. Mayrhofer defined "childbed fever" as a fermentation disease in which tissues decompose under the influence of living vibrions.[9] This meant that childbed fever could never occur without vibrions. By contrast, in the same year Mayrhofer delivered his final lecture, Gustav Braun—Carl Braun's brother and former student—published a book identifying the same range of causes Carl had listed in the 1850s.[10] By insisting on one necessary cause—a cause present in every case of childbed fever—Mayrhofer adopted the one central claim that distinguished Semmelweis's account from Braun's and from those of all of Semmelweis's other critics. Because Mayrhofer's concept of the disease focused on vibrions, his definition differed in content from the definition that Semmelweis had adopted, but his strategy of characterizing the disease in terms of a single universal cause was exactly the same.

It was immediately apparent that Mayrhofer's concept of the disease was closer to Semmelweis's than to Braun's. While Mayrhofer worked in the first section of the obstetrical clinic, Joseph Späth supervised the second section—the section in which midwives were trained. In 1863 and 1864 Späth published several statistical and historical studies of the incidence of childbed fever. In one such study, Späth wrote that Mayrhofer's discoveries confirmed Semmelweis's view because, according to Mayrhofer, the infective agents in the disease were vibrions that flourished in decomposed animal matter.[11] Späth also noted that, in spite of what may be said in public, every obstetrician now believed that Semmelweis had been correct.[12] Another Viennese obstetrician went even further: A. C. G. Veit wrote that, in addition to *confirming* Semmelweis's view, Mayrhofer and Späth had actually *refuted* Braun's opinion that ventilation significantly influenced the incidence of childbed fever.[13]

Contemporary physicians at the Viennese General Hospital were dismayed by the unusual bitterness manifested by advocates of the opposing theories of childbed fever.[14] By openly disagreeing with his chief, Mayrhofer sealed his own fate: his second lecture was poorly received, and, in spite of his initial success, Mayrhofer's work was rejected. Looking back a few years later, one contemporary physician observed, "If one says that Mayrhofer's work attracted universal attention, this should not be understood in one sense only. Such an energetic talent that transcends the mass of mediocrity often finds itself all too vulnerable."[15]

Soon after giving his second lecture, Mayrhofer left the first clinic and entered private practice. In 1870 he was appointed private docent of obstetrics and women's diseases, and a few years later he was appointed adjunct professor of the same specialty. At first, Mayrhofer met success in his private practice. However, through the 1870s, he experienced a series of misfortunes. While still working in the Viennese first clinic, Mayrhofer had suffered from lymphangitis and had begun to spit up blood. These symptoms indicated the onset of phthisis or tuberculosis, and in the nineteenth century, the disease was almost always fatal. As he entered private practice, his health continued to deteriorate. Then two of his children died. Mayrhofer also encountered frustrations in his medical practice. "The undeserved disappointments that Mayrhofer continued to experience soon drove him to morphine and lamed the vitality of this otherwise energetic individual."[16]

In 1878 Mayrhofer left Vienna. One contemporary ascribed the move to "a loss of interest in the affairs of practical life."[17] After a successful beginning in Tiflis (now Tbilisi in the Republic of Georgia), he moved to St. Petersburg, Russia, where he experienced further disappointments and frustrations. In 1881 he moved again, this time to the spa town of Franzensbad (now Franziskovy in the western end of the Czech Republic). During the following winter he became seriously ill. He died on 3 June 1882, one day after his forty-fifth birthday. A contemporary observed that "everyone who was close to Mayrhofer recognized that for him, death was a salvation."[18]

The striking parallels between Mayrhofer and Semmelweis have long been apparent. In a necrology, one nineteenth-century writer observed that Mayrhofer's "professional life was reminiscent of the tragic experiences of another gynecologist from the Vienna school, the genial Semmelweis."[19] In a book on the history of obstetrics in Vienna, I. Fischer notes that Mayrhofer's study of the role of germs in puerperal fever, which followed Pasteur's work and preceded Joseph Lister's, together with the circumstance that he was never properly appreciated in Vienna, earned him the title of a second Semmelweis.[20] Erna Lesky also refers to Mayrhofer as the second Semmelweis; in her book *The Vienna Medical School of the Nineteenth Century* she observes that Mayrhofer took up the problem of puerperal disease at the point at which Semmelweis had abandoned it.[21]

There has been a long-standing tradition that Semmelweis and Mayrhofer were generally ignored through the middle decades of the nineteenth century. While this was true in Austria and in Hungary, in Germany the situation was quite different.

Semmelweis's book was published in the fall of 1860. In 1861, at a meeting of German physicians and scientists, Wilhelm Lange, professor of obstetrics in Heidelberg, declared himself to be an adherent of Semmelweis's theory. Lange claimed that his own experiences and the mathematical basis of Semmelweis's work had persuaded him that Semmelweis was correct.[22] Between 1860 and 1865, the year in which Semmelweis died, Semmelweis's work was discussed in more than forty major medical publications and in more than a dozen reviews.[23] Most of these accounts appeared in German periodicals. Semmelweis, who had become preoccupied with past events, seems never to have realized that his ideas were being discussed and accepted in Germany.

In 1868, just three years after Semmelweis died, a German professor named Max Boehr noted that Semmelweis's theory of the infectious origin of childbed fever

> has the characteristic of every good pathological and physio-
> logical theory: it provides a unified, clear, and entirely
> intelligible meaning for a whole series of anatomical and
> clinical facts, and for the relevant experiences and discoveries
> of reliable observers of epidemics among maternity patients.
> None of the earlier or alternative theories or hypotheses
> regarding the occurrence of childbed fever has this char-
> acteristic to the same degree.[24]

Boehr believed Semmelweis's theory could account for every case of the disease. He observed that Semmelweis's work dealt a severe blow to "the superstitions of our predecessors, who believed in unknown cosmic-telluric-atmospheric influences and . . . in miasms."[25] Boehr mentioned that Veit, Späth, and Mayrhofer had supported Semmelweis's theory.

In the same year, Rudolf H. Ferber wrote that Semmelweis had initiated a revolution in the understanding of childbed fever. Ferber pointed out that "with only a few exceptions, the Semmelweis theory is now universally recognized in Germany."[26]

In 1876, Joseph Amann, professor of obstetrics in Munich, observed that Semmelweis's theory had become the shared property of the entire German medical profession.[27] Two years later, in 1878, another German physician observed that thirty-one years had passed "since Semmelweis first spoke the truth that every case of childbed fever comes about through the resorption of decaying animal-organic matter."[28] In the same year, Otto Spiegelberg, professor of medicine in Breslau, Germany, wrote that "Semmelweis deserves credit for placing the understanding of puerperal disease on the new and proper path." According to Spiegelberg, Semmelweis "explained that every case of puerperal fever is resorption fever, arising from the reception of decaying animal matter. . . . These claims hold today. In general, they contain everything there is to be said about puerperal fever."[29] Spiegelberg also credited Mayrhofer with having been the first to prove that puerperal fever was a parasitic process. Spiegelberg observed that once it had been clearly shown that puerperal fever was only a wound disease resting on a septic infection, this view "was rapidly accepted as common property, at least among the physicians in Germany."[30]

Until the 1870s, no important human disease had been conclusively traced to microorganisms, but there was a growing interest in establishing such a connection. In that decade, most physicians who studied the role of germs in disease etiology focused on infected wounds. This was true, in part, because every hospital contained patients suffering from wound infections, and such infections were easier to study than were internal disease processes. Moreover, the organic decomposition of infected wounds resembled fermentation, and Pasteur had shown that fermentation was always the result of living organisms that he called "ferments." This made it seem plausible that wound infections were due to living parasitic organisms. In the 1870s more than half of all publications associating bacteria with diseases concerned wound infections.[31] In the 1880s, both French and German physicians observed that the germ theory of disease had originated from studies of wound infections and especially from the investigation of childbed fever. Thus, while the Austrians and the Hungarians ignored Mayrhofer and seemed ashamed of Semmelweis's memory, elsewhere, their work was recognized and became part of the foundation for the modern germ theory of disease.

Through the nineteenth century, obstetricians gradually came to accept the views of Semmelweis and Mayrhofer, but, for tens of thousands of women, this acceptance came too late.

Sophia Jex-Blake, one of the first women to be awarded an M.D. degree in modern times, gave the following account of the origin of a childbed fever epidemic that occurred in Boston during the winter of 1866 and 1867:

> On *Friday, Nov 2nd*, A. S. was admitted to the Hospital and delivered of a female infant, which had apparently died two or three weeks previously. . . . A. S. was a married woman, but exhibited evident signs of syphilis, and to this infection the death *in utero* was probably due. On the following day, Saturday, one of the assistant doctors in the Hospital made a postmortem examination of the fetus, removing the uterus and other organs, and being thus occupied probably for some hours.
>
> On *Sunday, Nov 4th* K. M. entered the Hospital in the second stage of labor. Age 22; unmarried; primipara [first delivery]. . . . She had had labor pains to a greater or lesser extent, since the preceding Thursday, and, being homeless and friendless, she had been exposed to great hardships, and had, on the morning of her admission, walked into Boston from a distance, and then wandered about the streets for

hours before she was brought to the Hospital. It so happened that on her admission she was received and first examined by the assistant just mentioned, though subsequently delivered by another person. The baby . . . was born about 4 p.m., and a severe laceration of the perineum took place.[32]

Five days later, after great suffering, the woman died of child-bed fever, and over the next few weeks several other maternity patients died.

During the second half of the nineteenth century—in spite of the evidence generated by Semmelweis, Mayrhofer, and others—many doctors continued dissecting cadavers, examining patients, and arguing about etiology. Each year, oblivious to the suffering and tragedy by which they were engulfed, they consigned thousands of young women to early deaths.

Notes

1. Ignaz Semmelweis, *The Etiology, Concept, and Prophylaxis of Childbed Fever*, ed. and trans. K. Codell Carter (Madison: University of Wisconsin, 1983), pp. 246 f.

2. Carl Mayrhofer, ''Vorläufige Mittheilung über das Vorkommen von Vibrionen bei Wöchnerinnen und deren allfällige Bedeutung für Puerperaler krankungen,'' *Wochenblatt der Zeitschrift der k. k. Gesellschaft der Ärzte zu Wien* 19 (1863): 17–20, at p. 17

3. Mayerhofer, ''Vorläufige Mittheilung,'' p. 17.

4. Carl Mayrhofer, ''Untersuchungen über Aetiolgie der Puerperal-processe,'' *Zeitschrift der k. k. Gesellschaft der Ärzte zu Wien* 19 (1863): 28–42.

5. August Theodor Stamm, ''Ueber die Vernichtungsmöglichkeit des epidemischen Puerperalfiebers,'' *Wiener medizinische-Halle* 5 (1864). The essay appears in short segments between pages 157 and 477.

6. Carl Braun, ''Über Luftwechsel und Puerperalkrankheiten,'' *Wiener medizinische Wochenschrift* 14 (1864): cols. 257–259, and Carl Braum, ''Über Luftwechsel, den neuen Ventilations-Bau mit Benützung der natürlichen Temperaturdifferenzen und Luftströmung,'' *Medizinische Jahrbücher* 20 (1864): 165–208.

7. Carl Mayrhofer, ''Zur Frage nach der Ätiologie der Puerperalprocesse,'' *Monatschrift für Geburtskunde und Frauenkrankenheiten* 25 (1865): 112–134.

8. Carl Mayrhofer, *Sterilität des Weibes, Entwicklungsfehler und Entzündungen der Gebärmutter* (Stuttgart: Ferdinand Enke, 1882), p. 143.

9. Mayrhofer, ''Ätiologie der Puerperalprocesse,'' pp. 128, 134.

10. Gustav August Braun, *Compendium der Geburtshilfe* (Vienna: Braumüller, 1864), p. 305.

11. Josef Späth ''Statistische und historische Rückblicke auf die Vorkommnisse des Wiener Gebärhauses während der letzten dreissig Jahre mit besonderer Berücksichtigung der Puerperal-Erkrankungen,'' *Medizinische Jahrbücher* 20 (1864): 145–164, at p. 162.

12. Späth, ''Rückblicke,'' pp. 161 f.

13. A. C. G. Veit, ''Über die in der geburtshilflichen Klinik in Bonn im Sommer 1864 und Winter 1864–65 aufgetretenen puerperalen Erkrankungen,'' *Monatsschrift für Geburtskunde und Frauenkrankheiten* 26 (1865): 127–155, 161–208, at pp. 195 f.

14. Josef Späth, ''Über die Sanitäts-Verhältnisse der Wöchnerinnen an der Gebärklinik für Hebammen in Wien vom October 1861 bis Jänner 1863,'' *Medizinische Jahrbücher* 19 (1863): 10–27, at pp. 10–13.

15. An obituary notice of the death of Carl Mayrhofer, signed "r," *Wiener medizinische Blätter* 5 (1882): col. 725.

16. An obituary notice of the death of Carl Mayrhofer, signed "Ch.," *Wiener medizinische Presse* 23 (1882): cols. 778–779, at col. 779.

17. An obituary notice, *Wiener medizinische Presse*, col. 779.

18. An obituary notice, *Wiener medizinische Presse*, col. 779.

19. An obituary notice, *Wiener medizinische Presse*, col. 778.

20. I. Fischer, *Geschichte der Geburtshilfe in Wien* (Vienna: Vogel, 1909), p. 353.

21. Erna Lesky, *The Vienna Medical School of the Nineteenth Century* (Baltimore: Johns Hopkins, 1976), pp. 189 f.

22. Wilhelm Lange, "Semmelweiss'schen Theorie über die Entstehung des Puerperalfiebers," *Monatsschrift für Geburtskunde und Frauenkrankheiten* 18 (1861): 375 f.

23. K. Codell Carter, "Ignaz Semmelweis, Carl Mayrhofer, and the Rise of Germ Theory," *Medical History* 29 (1985): 33–53.

24. Max Boehr, "Über die Infectionstheorie des Puerperalfiebers und ihre Consequenzen für die Sanitäts-Polizei," *Monatsschrift für Geburtskunde und Frauenkrankheiten* 32 (1868): 401–433, at p. 403.

25. Boehr, p. 404.

26. Rudolf H. Ferber, "Die Ätiologie, Prophylaxis und Therapie des Puerperalfiebers," *Schmidt's Jahrbücher der Medizin* 139 (1868): 318–346, at p. 318.

27. Joseph Amann, *Klinik der Wochenbettkrankheiten* (Stuttgart: Ferdinand Enke, 1876), p. 67.

28. Brennecke, "Der puerperalfieber Frage," *Berliner klinische Wochenschrift* 16 (1878): 744–747, 758–761, at p. 744.

29. Otto Spiegelberg, *Lehrbuch der Geburtshülfe* (Lahr, Germany: Moritz Schauenburg, 1878), p. 714.

30. Otto Spiegelberg, "Die Entwicklung der puerperalen Infection," *Berliner klinische Wochenschrift* 17 (1880): 309–312, at p. 309.

31. Carter, p. 46.

32. Sophia Jex-Blake, "Puerperal Fever: An Inquiry into Its Nature and Treatment," M.D. diss., University of Bern, 1877, p. 23.

6

Puerperal Infection

What is the current medical concept of puerperal fever, and how common is the disease today? The U.S. Joint Committee on Maternal Welfare has defined "standard puerperal morbidity," as a "temperature of 100.4 [or higher], the temperature to occur in any two of the first ten days postpartum, exclusive of the first twenty-four hours, and to be taken by mouth by a standard technique at least four times daily."[1] A similar definition has been adopted in England: "a fever of 100.4 over a period of twenty-four or more hours during the three weeks after child-birth."[2] However, it is almost impossible to determine how frequently these standards are met. Women are usually discharged from maternity facilities within one to four days of delivery; and once they are discharged, no one regularly records their temperatures.

Moreover, even if one had such records, it is not clear exactly what they would reveal. An elevated temperature is not always a sign of morbidity. Fever is a common postpartum phenomenon, and it can have various causes, such as hormonal changes, reaction to drugs, or various medical conditions unrelated to delivery. Most postpartum fevers subside spontaneously within a few days and have no adverse consequences, so they may not really indicate puerperal morbidity. As nineteenth-century physicians often observed, not all fever in puerperae is puerperal fever.

At present, medicine favors concepts of diseases that describe either an observable change in body tissues or the cause of symptoms. These preferences reflect the influence of pathological anatomy and of the quest for causal definitions. Thus, the concept of ''puerperal fever'' is no longer favored as a diagnostic category. In its place, modern medical texts employ two kinds of terms. First, as was the case in the nineteenth century, it is common to identify the specific organs or tissues that are changed in puerperal disease. For this purpose, physicians use such terms as ''endometritis'' (inflammation of the mucous membrane of the uterus), ''metrophlebitis'' (inflammation of the veins of the uterus), and ''peritonitis'' (inflammation of the serous membrane that lines the walls of the abdomen)—terms invented by eighteenth- and nineteenth-century pathologists. However, there is this difference: in the nineteenth century, these terms simply identified inflammations in particular tissues and were strictly neutral with respect to causation; today, the use of a term like ''endometritis'' often presupposes that the inflammation in the specified tissue is due to an infection by parasitic microorganisms.

Second, in place of the term ''puerperal fever,'' physicians also speak of infection, sepsis, shock, or toxicity. These terms differ from terms like ''metrophlebitis'' or ''peritonitis'' in that they give no indication where the disease process is focused. They also differ from terms like ''fever'' or ''inflammation'' in that they name different ways in which fever and other observable signs and symptoms originate. In this latter sense, each of these concepts is at least partially causal. ''Infection'' is any abnormal multiplication of parasitic organisms in a living host, and ''sepsis'' is the destruction of living tissues by parasitic organisms. Thus, these terms are closely related. ''Shock'' refers to a sudden reduction in the volume of blood returning to the heart from the peripheral circulatory system. Shock can be caused by different conditions, such as hemorrhage or allergy, but it can also be caused by infection. "Toxicity" refers to the accumulation of toxins or poisons within the body; this also can have various causes, one of which is infection. Thus, in the context of puerperal morbidity, while infection, sepsis, shock, and toxicity are distinguishable conditions, they occur regularly in combination. The earlier concept of puerperal fever included many, but not all, of the cases that would now fall into each of these categories. The modern terms used most commonly in reference to what earlier physicians would have called "childbed fever" are "puerperal infection" and "puerperal sepsis."

However, in using these two modern terms, one must be careful not to introduce an ambiguity. Both terms could be taken to refer to some condition in puerperae that is either unrelated or only indirectly related to delivery. For example, urinary tract infections are fifteen times more common in women than in men, and the incidence of such infections increases during pregnancy. One could refer to a urinary tract infection in puerperae as a puerperal infection. However, using the term so broadly would reduce its usefulness and would also be inconsistent with the historical context from which the term has emerged. Insofar as they were able, nineteenth-century physicians would have excluded these cases from their category of "childbed fever," and this is also done today. Thus, "puerperal infection" and "puerperal sepsis" are usually limited to genital tract infections that follow and result from labor, delivery, or abortion; this is the sense in which we will use these terms.

How common is puerperal infection? A study conducted in 1951 at Queen Charlotte's Hospital in London found that of 2,701 deliveries there were 1,423 cases of fever but only 141 cases— just over 0.5 percent of the total births—of "true genital tract infections."[3] However, many physicians routinely prescribe prophylactic antibiotics to all puerperae, and antibiotics are always administered promptly to any patient who seems especially at risk.

Thus, many incipient puerperal infections are controlled before they become clinically apparent, and the 1951 study is not a reliable indication of the true incidence of such infections. Obviously it would be unconscionable to withhold treatment for the sole purpose of determining the ordinary frequency of infection; therefore, one must be content with estimates. In the United States at the present time, puerperal infection is believed to occur in between 1 and 8 percent of all deliveries,[4] a rate close to the incidence of puerperal fever reported in successful nineteenth-century maternity facilities. On the other hand, in the United States at the present time, only about one hundred women die each year from puerperal sepsis—about three for every one hundred thousand deliveries. This rate of mortality—although a substantial part of the overall rate of maternal mortality and a terrible burden—would be regarded by nineteenth-century obstetricians as incredibly favorable.

Today, the single most important risk factor for puerperal infection is cesarean section.

> Both for frequency and severity of pelvic infection, cesarean section has emerged in the last few decades as the major predisposing clinical factor. . . . [Cesarean section involves] a five to thirty fold increase in risk of puerperal infection. Published accounts of post cesarean section infection reveal that endometritis occurs in twelve to fifty-one percent. . . . Bacteremia develops in eight to twenty percent, and other serious complications . . . occur in two to four percent of indigent patients with endometritis after cesarean section. . . . Reasons for higher infection after cesarean section include increased intrauterine manipulation, foreign body (suture material), tissue necrosis at the suture line, hematomaseroma formation, and wound infection.[5]

Another important risk factor for puerperal sepsis is socioeconomic status: indigent women have higher than normal rates of infection.

The rates may be higher because these women are more likely to deliver in teaching hospitals, where they are examined more frequently during labor. In other words, as in Semmelweis's day, their increased risk stems not from a lack of medical attention, but from too much of it.

Other risk factors include the frequency of vaginal examinations, the level of fetal monitoring, and the length of stay in hospitals. As in the past, most of today's risk factors for puerperal infection involve forms of medical intervention. Other things being equal, the less the medical involvement in the birth process and the shorter the patient's stay in the hospital, the healthier she is likely to be.

Within thirty years of the publication of Semmelweis's *Etiology of Childbed Fever*, physicians had concluded that microorganisms—rather than decaying organic matter—caused what was then called "childbed fever." By the late 1880s, physicians had concluded that a particular kind of microorganism—streptococci—were most frequently involved in the disease. Which microorganisms are now regarded as the causes of puerperal sepsis?

Postpartum genital tract infections ordinarily involve a variety of organisms; in most cases, there is no one causal agent. In a recent study, more than 80 percent of cases of puerperal endometritis were found to involve more than one species of organism. On average, about three different organisms would be identified in each case of the disease.[6]

At any given moment, the human body is inhabited by billions of microorganisms. Those that regularly inhabit the body are called "endogenous"; those that invade opportunistically are called "exogenous." Usually, both kinds of organisms are relatively harmless, and many endogenous organisms actually contribute to good health in various ways. The body's defenses repel most invasions of potentially pathogenic organisms before they cause observable disease symptoms. Even many infections of streptococcal bacilli have no harmful consequences. On average, people experience symptomatic disease episodes caused by streptococci about every three to four years, and asymptomatic infections are even more common.

As a part of their ordinary metabolic processes, microorganisms create various chemical byproducts that are either given off as waste or become incorporated into the structure of the parasite. Metabolic wastes diffuse more or less randomly through the tissues surrounding the parasite; and while some of these byproducts are harmless, metabolic wastes and even parts of the microorganism itself can be poisonous to the host. Some metabolic wastes from microorganisms are exceptionally virulent. Indeed, they include the most deadly of any known poisons: for instance, "it has been calculated that as little as seven ounces of crystalline botulinum type A toxin would suffice to kill the entire human population of the world."[7] When pathogenic parasites multiply within the body, the toxins they generate may become so abundant in the living tissues that they gradually poison the host. The result is what we call "disease." At present, it is not possible to trace each specific disease symptom to the production of a specific toxin. However, most of the symptoms associated with ordinary infectious diseases are assumed to result from this process of intoxication.

Streptococci are unable to produce for themselves all the vitamins and amino acids that they require, and these nutrients must ordinarily be derived by breaking down the host's tissues. For this reason, streptococci cannot easily be grown outside living animals. However, in the late nineteenth century, researchers found that streptococci could flourish on a combination of sheep blood and agar; this red opaque gelatin came into common use as a culture medium. When streptococci grow on blood agar, some colonies become surrounded by a greenish margin while others form a margin that is transparent. When examined under a microscope, agar from the greenish margins can be seen to contain many discolored blood corpuscles, whereas agar from transparent margins contains no blood corpuscles at all. This is interpreted to mean that the streptococci that form greenish margins are unable to disintegrate completely the red blood cells embedded in the agar, while those that form transparent margins are able to do so. In 1903 Hugo Schottmuller proposed using this difference as a basis for classifying streptococci. Strains of organisms that form greenish margins on blood agar are called "alpha-hemolytic," and those that produce clear margins are called "beta-hemolytic" or, frequently, just "hemolytic." Still other strains produce no visible changes in blood agar, and these strains are called "gamma-hemolytic." All three varieties can cause human and animal diseases, but the overwhelming majority of all pathogenic streptococci are beta-hemolytic.

Streptococci are also classified in terms of the immune reactions that they provoke when they invade a new host, and this classification cuts across the classification in terms of hemolytic reactions. When an alien substance is introduced into living tissues, the immune system may begin producing distinctive molecules that become attached to the alien ones just introduced. Alien substances that trigger this response in the immune system are called "antigens," and the molecules produced by the immune system are called "antibodies." By becoming attached to an antigen, the antibody helps reduce its harmful effect on the body. This can be accomplished in various ways. Some antibodies group antigens into clumps so that they cannot diffuse through the body; some mark antigens for subsequent destruction by other components of the immune system; and other antibodies merely coat antigens so that the host is shielded from their toxic effects. For the most part, each antibody is created specifically to attack one particular kind of antigen, so new antibodies must be created each time the body is invaded by antigens of a new kind.

In reality, streptococci and other bacteria are enormous in comparison to the size of individual antigenic molecules; and instead of treating an invading bacterium as a single antigen, the immune system typically produces a variety of antibodies that attach themselves to various specific parts of the cell walls of the invaders. Thus, different segments of the cell walls of a given bacterium may function as different antigens and provoke the production of different antibodies. The cell walls of streptococcal bacilli contain particular carbohydrate molecules that function as antigens. In 1933 the American bacteriologist Rebecca C. Lancefield proposed classifying streptococci according to the antigenic properties of these carbohydrates. She originally distinguished five main groups of bacilli, which she labeled by the letters A through E.

Lancefield found that the streptococci recovered from most human infections were included in her group A. She originally isolated from cattle the bacilli that constituted group B. Group C strains came from various animals such as cattle, horses, rabbits, and guinea pigs. Group D organisms came from cheese, and group E streptococci were isolated from milk.[8] Two years later, Lancefield and Ronald Hare identified two new groups, F and G. They also reported research on the incidence of different groups of streptococci in infections of the birth canal of postpartum women. They noted that

> the vast majority of strains from definite infections of the uterus are members of group A. . . . The vast majority of hemolytic streptococci from the birth canal which do not bring about active infections are not members of this group. Most of them fall either into group B or D. . . . The human nasopharynx is the main reservoir of group A strains in nature. Because of this, and because of the great rarity of group A streptococci in the normal vagina, *ante partum*, there can be little doubt that the vast majority of puerperal hemolytic streptococci infections are due to inoculation from some other source than the patient's genital tract and probably arise from the above mentioned reservoir in the patient or attendants.[9]

This was an important discovery. In the 1930s, obstetricians believed that puerperal sepsis was ordinarily due to streptococci that were endogenous to the birth canal. This meant that the physicians themselves were not responsible for most cases of the disease and that they could do little or nothing to prevent it. Of course, this was a slightly more sophisticated version of the same general attitude that Semmelweis had opposed seventy years earlier. And as in Semmelweis's time, this belief fostered carelessness in the use of antiseptic measures. It was generally believed that obstetrical operations—such as delivery—required less stringent antiseptic measures than were required in surgery.[10] Lancefield's discovery that puerperal sepsis is usually caused by group A streptococci conclusively refuted this view and proved *once again* that most cases of puerperal infection were caused by the intervention of medical personnel.

Within Lancefield's classification scheme, which is still in use today, group A streptococci are recognized as the most important bacterial agents in human disease. Consequently, organisms of this group have been studied extensively. Group A bacilli seem to form two natural classes: strains from one class usually attack the skin, and strains from the other class attack the throat. Group A strains that cause skin infections are more common in warm climates, they seem not to occur epidemically, and they usually cause local rather than systemic disease symptoms. By contrast, group A strains that typically invade the throat are more common in cold climates and in the winter, they often occur in epidemics, and they frequently cause systemic symptoms such as fever. If allowed to invade the body under suitable conditions, group A strains of this second variety can also cause such diseases as erysipelas, pneumonia, rheumatic fever, scarlet fever, and puerperal fever.

Most of the horrible epidemics of childbed fever in the eighteenth and nineteenth centuries were probably caused by those strains of group A streptococcal bacilli that normally attack the throat. This conjecture is based on clinical, pathological, and epidemiological similarities between what was reported in the great epidemics and modern observations of disease episodes known to be caused by these group A bacilli.

In contrast to group A organisms, group B streptococci are often endogenous to healthy humans; they are commonly found in the intestinal tract and in the female genitals. Between 5 and 30 percent of pregnant women have vaginal colonies of group B streptococci, and the rate seems to be highest for Caucasian women under twenty years of age. These bacilli can spread to the urinary tract, where they can cause infections.

In 1935, R. M. Fry reported finding group B bacilli in three cases of puerperal sepsis.[11] However, during the next three decades, group B streptococci received little medical attention. Reports of group B infections became more common in the medical literature during the 1960s; and in succeeding decades, such reports have become ever more prominent. Puerperal infections from endogenous group B strep usually occur when the genitals are damaged in delivery and the organisms invade the bloodstream or other tissues. Patients undergoing cesarean section are particularly at risk. Postpartum group B streptococcal infections typically involve the sudden onset of high fever, usually within twelve hours after delivery. However, the symptoms in group B infections are sometimes indistinguishable from those observed in group A infections, and conclusive identification of the causal agent requires bacteriological examination. Whether the increase in reported cases reflects a shift in the relative prevalence of the causal agents themselves or whether the change is to be explained in some other way remains to be seen.

In spite of the great notoriety of the puerperal fever epidemics in earlier centuries, sporadic cases of the disease have probably always accounted for at least as many total deaths as have the epidemics.[12] On the other hand, since the epidemics were mostly limited to the inhabitants of maternity clinics, sporadic cases are drawn from a larger population. Thus, while they may account for more total deaths, they are proportionately less common. That many sporadic cases were caused by endogenous group B streptococci that exploited an opportunity to invade the damaged genital tissues of the puerperae now seems likely. These cases would explain many of the instances Semmelweis attributed to self-infection.

In the context of human birth, there is one striking difference between group A and group B infections. Group A streptococci generally attack the mother, usually when exogenous bacilli are introduced into the birth canal by medical attendants. By contrast, group B infections generally attack the fetus or the neonate when it is exposed to bacilli that are either endogenous to the birth canal or else carried by medical personnel. About 75 percent of babies delivered by women who harbor vaginal group B streptococci become contaminated in the course of delivery; however, only a small percentage of these babies become diseased. Moreover, between 16 and 45 percent of nursery personnel carry group B streptococci, and contamination of the newborn by medical attendants is also very common.

Altogether it has been estimated that twelve thousand to fifteen thousand newborns contract group B streptococcal infections each year and that within this group the mortality rate is about 50 percent.[13] A German study conducted between 1983 and 1988 examined 222 cases of neonatal septicemia and meningitis. The incidence of disease was just below 1 percent of all the babies delivered; and of those who became ill, the fatality rate was 45.9 percent. Group B streptococci were frequently isolated as one of the causal agents. Following criteria established by the U.S. Centers for Disease Control in Atlanta, these German researchers concluded that ''152 (68.5%) of the 222 infections were nosocomial.''[14] The term ''nosocomial'' refers to a condition contracted within the hospital environment. So the conclusion of this study is that well over half of all the neonates who became diseased had contracted their infections from their hospital surroundings.

There is also evidence that the rate of group B infection among neonates is increasing. A recent Swedish study found that the rate of neonatal group B infections increased consistently between 1973 and 1985. The authors concluded that the increase "probably reflects a true increment related to an increased rate of colonization of pregnant women with GBS [group B streptococci] during this period."[15] So group B streptococci present a real and growing threat to the health of mothers and especially of infants.

Streptococci from groups C and G are also found in the female genital tract, and both have been associated with epidemic and sporadic puerperal sepsis.[16] However, these are not common pathogens in puerperal disease.

In addition to streptococci, several other parasitic organisms can cause puerperal infections. From the middle of the nineteenth century, it has been recognized that many organisms— including streptococci—flourish in the presence of ordinary air while others can survive only in atmospheres that contain little free oxygen. The former are called "aerobic" and the latter "anaerobic." Various anaerobic microorganisms are normally endogenous to the female genitals. During the latter part of the nineteenth century, researchers established that various other anaerobic organisms could invade the human body opportunistically and cause different infections. Anaerobic organisms have probably accounted for a significant percentage of sporadic cases of puerperal infection.[17]

Escherichia coli, commonly known as *E. coli*, is an aerobic bacterium that normally flourishes harmlessly in the intestinal tract. However, when *E. coli* invades other tissues, it can cause several serious diseases, including gastric disorders among the newborn, urinary tract infections in adults, and puerperal sepsis. *E. coli* is readily spread by the bloodstream and can cause infections throughout the body. *E. coli* invasions of the vascular system are characterized by the sudden onset of alternating fever and chills, and, by a process not yet understood, such infections are usually accompanied by shock. Indeed, *E. coli* is the most common cause of puerperal septic shock.[18]

How effectively can puerperal sepsis be controlled by prophylactic cleanliness? Even in the last two decades of the nineteenth century there was good evidence that streptococci were the most common cause of childbed fever. One would expect this knowledge to have prompted the use of antiseptic measures that would have significantly reduced the incidence of infection. Yet, surprisingly, recognition of the causal agents seems to have had almost no impact on maternal mortality. In 1910, Arnold Lea of Manchester observed,

> In the five years 1851–5 the puerperal death rate from all causes [in England and Wales] was 4.9 per 1000 [births], and in the five years ending 1906 it still amounted to 4.2 per thousand. . . . [We] do no violence to the statistics if we put down the septic [puerperal fever] mortality in England and Wales at between 3000 and 5000 per annum.[19]

Maternal mortality remained essentially constant through the next twenty-five years. As Irvine Loudon has pointed out, any decline in morbidity probably resulted from a reduction in the virulence of the streptococci themselves or from a decrease in availability of the organisms in the population at large, rather than from improvements in medical practice.[20]

One reason for the persisting mortality rate was that until Lancefield proved puerperal sepsis was usually exogenous, obstetricians saw little reason to adhere to strict aseptic and antiseptic standards. So they continued to infect their patients. Another reason that mortality remained so high was the inherent difficulty of preventing infection by antiseptic measures alone. Once a person has been colonized by streptococci, he or she may continue to carry and to spread pathogenic organisms for weeks, months, or even years—certainly long after all symptoms have disappeared. Moreover, many and possibly most cases of strep infection are asymptomatic. Thus, at any given time, a significant percentage of the population may be carrying and spreading group A streptococci without even knowing that they are infected.

> Following an epidemic that attacked twenty women in the Boston hospital in 1965, epidemiologists found that about five percent of the hospital staff and ten to fifteen percent of the neighboring community were asymptomatic carriers of hemolytic streptococci. Of the forty hospital carriers, four had positive throat cultures for group A and one had a positive skin lesion.[21]

Even if medical personnel were to wash conscientiously, many of them would be carrying group A streptococci in their noses and throats at any given time. From these sources they could constantly reinfect their hands. Moreover, the patients and visitors who enter delivery facilities may also carry streptococci. After delivery, patients can sometimes infect themselves or each other, or they can be infected by visitors.

Streptococci are usually spread by touching, but they can also be spread through the air by way of dust particles, called "fomites." It is not known how readily streptococci can be carried by fomites, and currently most hospitals give relatively little attention to this problem.

> Current infectious disease officers recommend a hospital practice that places less emphasis on the control of fomites and more emphasis on the isolation of carriers and the washing of hands between patients. This is designed to prevent the direct transmission of infection from patient to patient and from attendant to patient.[22]

But even if fomites are not the usual means by which infection is conveyed, such a conveyance can occur. Taking all of this into account, it is unlikely that even conscientious washing of the kind that Semmelweis recommended could, by itself, prevent dissemination of the causal organisms. At least given present opinion, the control of puerperal sepsis depends at least as much on therapy as on prophylactic cleanliness.

Irvine Loudon has shown that 1937 was the crucial year in which chemotherapy first significantly reduced maternal mortality. While it is possible that the decline in mortality was due, in part, to a spontaneous reduction in the virulence of streptococci, the decline seems to have been due primarily to the introduction of a class of drugs known as "sulfonamides."[23]

In 1932 a group of German chemists working at an industrial laboratory synthesized various chemical compounds in the quest for an antibacterial agent that could be taken internally. One of the chemicals they produced was called "prontosil." In 1935 a member of this group, Gerhard Domagk, announced that prontosil—although relatively ineffective against bacteria grown experimentally outside the body—protected living mice against virulent streptococci. Four years later in 1939, Domagk was awarded the Nobel prize for his work; but by that time the National Socialists (the Nazis) controlled Germany, and Domagk was obliged to refuse the award.

Shortly after the announcement of Domagk's discovery, French chemists showed that the specific part of the complex prontosil molecule that was effective against streptococci was an aminophenyl-sulfamide and that other related chemicals built from this same constituent could also be useful.

Over the next few months, various physicians reported the use of prontosil on humans suffering from erysipelas and from puerperal fever. The reports were consistently favorable but were accompanied by too little clinical and bacteriological evidence to be really conclusive. In 1936 Leonard Colebrook and Meave Kenny published two reports of trials using prontosil on mice and on a total of sixty-four victims of puerperal sepsis. Prontosil was found to be effective even in advanced cases in which streptococci could be readily isolated from the patient's blood—a condition that, in most instances, "made the prognosis extremely grave."[24] One very ill patient had a temperature of 105 degrees, and each cubic centimeter of her blood produced more than five thousand colonies of hemolytic streptococci. Colebrook noted that previously he had found bacilli concentrations of this magnitude only in terminal stages of fatal infections. Yet, incredibly, on the fourth day of treatment, the patient's blood was sterile and her temperature had fallen to the normal level. Although he tried to be appropriately cautious in reporting his work, Colebrook could only describe the effects of prontosil as spectacular. This was the first time any chemotherapy had been proven effective against streptococci. Within months, the sulfonamides were being so widely used that, even in the first year of their use, they significantly reduced maternal mortality in the British Isles.

However, the use of prontosil and of the other sulfonamides was subject to various problems. Strains of hemolytic streptococci soon emerged that were resistant to treatment by these drugs, and patients sometimes developed allergic reactions. There was clearly a need for other drugs that would be more effective and yet less toxic.

The discovery of penicillin by Alexander Fleming in 1928 (along with its subsequent development in the 1940s) was destined to have a greater impact on the treatment of streptococcal infections than any other single therapeutic measure before or since. Fleming made his initial discovery when airborne mold spores accidentally invaded a culture plate and began growing among colonies of the staphylococci that Fleming was cultivating. Fleming noticed that the bacilli colonies surrounding the mold disintegrated spontaneously. He removed the mold and cultivated it in a new medium. He then brushed streaks of different pathogens across the new mold cultures. As had happened with the colonies of staph, many of the new pathogens were destroyed by the mold. Fleming identified the mold as a variety of *Penicillium*, and he demonstrated that the active substance, which he named "penicillin," was not toxic to humans. Fleming tried to concentrate and to purify penicillin but could produce only an unstable liquid unsuitable for medical purposes.

The development of the sulfonamides in the late 1930s stimulated interest in chemotherapy generally and provided the incentive to renew the investigation of penicillin. A group of Oxford chemists, especially Howard Walter Florey and Ernst Boris Chain, managed to concentrate penicillin and to produce from it a stable and solid substance that could be used medically. During the early 1940s, they also conducted animal trials showing that penicillin was not toxic to animals but was very effective against a wide range of pathogens. The results of the first human trials were published in 1941. Four years later in 1945, Fleming, Florey, and Chain were awarded a Nobel prize for their discoveries.

Penicillin and its numerous derivatives are generally effective against group A streptococci, and they remain the drugs of choice for dealing with most cases of puerperal sepsis. However, as we have seen, puerperal sepsis is usually a polymicrobial infection, and some of the possible causal agents—for example, group B streptococci—are not always fully responsive to penicillin therapy. For this reason, at present, puerperal sepsis is usually treated with a combination of different antibiotics.

Chemotherapy is successful in most cases, but serious problems remain: First, some patients continue to die or to suffer serious disabilities either in spite of the therapy or sometimes because of complications arising directly or indirectly from the therapy. Second, microorganisms change rapidly, and there is good evidence that their levels of virulence have fluctuated significantly during the past two or three centuries. There is also evidence that new and more virulent strains of group A streptococci may now be emerging.[25] But whether or not this proves to be true, the possibility remains a constant threat. Third, in many cases the virulence of microorganisms is associated with ethnic and economic conditions; modern antibiotics have been less successful in controlling puerperal sepsis in non-Western cultures than in Europe and America. For these reasons, puerperal sepsis remains a formidable threat both to delivering women and to neonates throughout the world.

Notes

1. Ronald S. Gibbs and Richard L. Sweet, "Maternal and Fetal Infections," in Robert K. Creasy and Robert Resnik, *Maternal and Fetal Medicine Principles and Practice*, pp. 603–678 (Philadelphia: W. B. Saunders, 1984), at p. 622.

2. Margaret DeLacy, "Puerperal Fever in Eighteenth-Century Britain," *Bulletin of the History of Medicine* 63 (1989): 521–556, at p. 524.

3. DeLacy, p. 524.

4. Gibbs and Sweet, p. 623.

5. Gibbs and Sweet, p. 623.

6. D. Heather Watts et al., "Early Postpartum Endometritis: The Role of Bacteria, Genital Mycoplasmas, and *Chlamydia trachomatis*," *Obstetrics and Gynaecology* 73 (1989): 52–60, at p. 58.

7. Bob A. Freeman, *Burrows Textbook of Microbiology*, 21st ed. (Philadelphia: W. B. Saunders, 1979), p. 226.

8. Rebecca C. Lancefield, "A Serological Differentiation of Human and Other Groups of Hemolytic Streptococci," *Journal of Experimental Medicine* 57 (1933): 571–595.

9. Rebecca C. Lancefield and Ronald Hare, "The Serological Differentiation of Pathogenic and Non-pathogenic Strains of Hemolytic Streptococci from Parturient Women," *Journal of Experimental Medicine* 61 (1935): 347.

10. Irvine Loudon, "Puerperal Fever, the Streptococcus, and the Sulfonamides, 1911–1945," *British Medical Journal* 295 (1987): 485–490, at p. 487.

11. R. M. Fry, "Fatal Infection by Hemolytic Streptococci Group B," *Lancet* 1 (1938): 199.

12. Edward Shorter, *A History of Women's Bodies* (London: Allen Lane, 1983), chapter 6.

13. Gibbs and Sweet, p. 632.

14. E. L. Grauel et al., "Neonatal Septicaemia—Incidence, Etiology, and Outcome," *Acta Paediatrica Scandinavica* 360, Supplement (1989): 113–119, at pp. 117 f.

15. I. Sjöberg et al., "Incidence of Early Onset Group B Streptococcal Septicemia in Sweden 1973–1985," *European Journal of Clinical Microbiology and Infectious Diseases* 9 (1990): 276–278, at p. 277.

16. Isaac Ginsburg, "Streptococcus," in Abraham I. Braude, Charles E. Davis, and Joshua Fierer, *Infectious Diseases and Medical Microbiology*, 2nd ed., pp. 242–253 (Philadelphia: W. B. Saunders, 1986), at p. 250.

17. Stanley A. Seligman, "The Lesser Pestilence: Non-epidemic Puerperal Fever," *Medical History* 35 (1991): 89–102.

18. Gibbs and Sweet, p. 627.

19. Quoted in Loudon, p. 485.

20. Louden, p. 485.

21. DeLacy, pp. 527 f.

22. DeLacy, pp. 528 f.

23. Loudon, p. 485.

24. Leonard Colebrook and Meave Kenny, ''Treatment of Human Puerperal Infections and of Experimental Infections in Mice, with Prontosil,'' *Lancet* 1 (1936): 1279–1286; Leonard Colebrook and Meave Kenny, ''Treatment with Prontosil of Puerperal Infections Due to Hemolytic Streptococci,'' *Lancet* 2 (1936): 1319–1322.

25. Seligman, p. 92.

Postscript

Knowledge does not come without cost. Three centuries elapsed between the first epidemic of childbed fever and the discovery of penicillin. For three hundred years, physicians examined young women in childbirth, watched them die, dissected their corpses, and deposited their remains in unmarked graves. The doctors gained knowledge, but at the sacrifice of more lives than were lost in all the wars of those centuries.

In towns and villages around the world are memorials that preserve, in honored glory, the names of men who died at war—men who, in hatred, killed one another, for causes that now seem empty and vain. But there are no memorials to the victims of childbed fever. We remember them no more, and their names are lost forever. Yet their sacrifice purchased knowledge that blesses all our lives with increased health and security.

Never have blessings been sanctified by the payment of so terrible a price. Never have the beneficiaries of such blessings been so oblivious of the cost and of those who paid it.

Selected Bibliography

Arneth, Franz Hektor. "Evidence of Puerperal Fever depending on the Contagious Inoculation of Morbid Matter." *Monthly Journal of Medical Science* 12 (1851): 505–511.

Benedek, István. *Ignaz Philipp Semmelweis*. Vienna: Hermann Böhlaus, 1983.

_____. *Semmelweis' Krankheit*. Budapest, Hungary: Akadémiai Kiadó, 1983.

Carter, K. Codell. "On the Decline of Bloodletting in Nineteenth-Century Medicine." *Journal of Psychoanalytic Anthropology* 5 (1982): 219–234.

_____, ed. and trans. *Essays of Robert Koch*. Westport, CT: Greenwood Press, 1987.

_____. "Ignaz Semmelweis, Carl Mayrhofer, and the Rise of Germ Theory." *Medical History* 29 (1985): 33–53.

_____. "Josef Skoda's Relation to the Work of Ignaz Semmelweis." *Medizinhistorisches Journal* 19 (1984): 335–347.

_____. "Semmelweis and His Predecessors." *Medical History* 25 (1981): 57–72.

_____, Scott Abbott, and James L. Siebach. "Five Documents Relating to the Final Illness and Death of Ignaz Semmelweis." *Bulletin of the History of Medicine*, forthcoming.

_____, and George S. Tate. "The Earliest-Known Account of Semmelweis's Initiation of Disinfection at Vienna's Allgemeines Krankenhaus." *Bulletin of the History of Medicine* 65 (1991): 252–257.

Churchill, Fleetwood, ed. *Essays on the Puerperal Fever*. London: Sydenham Society, 1849.

Colebrook, Leonard, and Meave Kenny. "Treatment of Human Puerperal Infections, and of Experimental Infections in Mice, with Prontosil." *Lancet* 1 (1936): 1279–1286.

————. "Treatment with Prontosil of Puerperal Infections Due to Hemolytic Streptococci." *Lancet* 2 (1936): 1319–1322.

DeLacy, Margaret. "Puerperal Fever in Eighteenth-Century Britain." *Bulletin of the History of Medicine* 63 (1989): 521–556.

Fischer, I. *Geschichte der Geburtshilfe in Wien.* Vienna: Vogel, 1909.

Gerster. "Das medicinische Wien." *Archiv für physiologische Heilkunde* 6 (1847): 320–329, 468–480.

Gibbs, Ronald S., and Richard L. Sweet. "Maternal and Fetal Infections." In Robert K. Creasy and Robert Resnik, *Maternal and Fetal Medicine Principles and Practice,* 603–678. Philadelphia: W. B. Saunders, 1984.

Gortvay, György, and Imre Zoltán. *Semmelweis: His Life and Work.* Budapest, Hungary: Akadémiai Kiadó, 1968.

Grauel, E. L., et al. "Neonatal Septicaemia—Incidence, Etiology, and Outcome." *Acta Paediatrica Scandinavica* 360, Supplement (1989): 113–119.

Jetter, Dieter. *Wien von den Anfängen bis um 1900.* Vol. 5 of Geschichte des Hospitals. Wiesbaden, Germany: Franz Steiner, 1982.

Jex-Blake, Sophia. "Puerperal Fever: An Inquiry into Its Nature and Treatment." M.D. diss., University of Bern, 1877.

Lancefield, Rebecca C. "A Serological Differentiation of Human and Other Groups of Hemolytic Streptococci." *Journal of Experimental Medicine* 57 (1933): 571–595.

————, and Ronald Hare. "The Serological Differentiation of Pathogenic and Non-pathogenic Strains of Hemolytic Streptococci from Parturient Women." *Journal of Experimental Medicine* 61 (1935): 347.

Lesky, Erna. *Ignaz Philipp Semmelweis und die Wiener medizinische Schule.* Vienna: Hermann Böhlaus, 1964.

————. *Meilensteine der Wiener Medizin.* Vienna: Wilhelm Maudrich, 1981.

————. *The Vienna Medical School of the Nineteenth Century.* Baltimore: Johns Hopkins, 1976.

Loudon, Irvine. "Puerperal Fever, the Streptococcus, and the Sulfonamides, 1911–1945." *British Medical Journal* 295 (1987): 485–490.

Murphy, Frank P. "Ignaz Philipp Semmelweis: An Annotated Bibliography." *Bulletin of the History of Medicine* 20 (1946): 653–707.

Routh, C. H. F. "On the Causes of the Endemic Puerperal Fever of Vienna." *Medico-chirurgical Transactions* 32 (1849): 27–40.

Seligman, Stanley A. "The Lesser Pestilence: Non-epidemic Puerperal Fever." *Medical History* 35 (1991): 89–102.

Semmelweis, Ignaz. *The Etiology, Concept, and Prophylaxis of Childbed Fever.* Ed. and trans. K. Codell Carter. Madison: University of Wisconsin, 1983.

Shorter, Edward. *A History of Women's Bodies.* London: Allen Lane, 1983.

Silló-Seidl, Georg. *Die Wahrheit über Semmelweis.* Geneva, Switzerland: Ariston, 1978.

Thomas, Robert. *The Modern Practice of Physic.* 8th ed. London: Longman, 1825.

Von Györy, Tiberius. *Semmelweis' gesammelte Werke.* Jena, Germany: Gustav Fischer, 1905.

Watts, Heather, et al. "Early Postpartum Endometritis: The Role of Bacteria, Genital Mycoplasmas, and *Chlamydia trachomatis.*" *Obstetrics and Gynaecology* 73 (1989): 52–60.

White, Charles. *A Treatise on the Management of Pregnant and Lying-in Women.* London: E. and C. Dilly, 1773.

Wilson, T. G. *Victorian Doctor: Being the Life of Sir William Wilde.* London: Methuen, 1942.

Index